Medical School Professors
Reveal

The
Science And Art
Of
Living A Longer
And
Healthier Life

CHARTING A COURSE FOR THE NEW MILLENNIUM

By

CARL E. BARTECCHI, M.D.
and
ROBERT W. SCHRIER, M.D.

Foreword by Richard D. Lamm
Governor of Colorado (1975-1987)
Quotations sourced by
Barbara Lindley Schrier

EMIS, Inc.
Medical Publishers
Durant, Oklahoma

ISBN: 0-917634-04-7

Library of Congress Cataloging-in-Publication Data

Bartecchi, Carl E.
  Medical school professors reveal the science and art of living a longer and healthier life : charting a course for the new millennium / by Carl E. Bartecchi and Robert W. Schrier ; foreword by Richard D. Lamm ; quotations sourced by Barbara Lindley Schrier.
    p. cm.
  Includes bibliographical references.
  ISBN 0-917634-04-7 (pbk.)
    1. Health--Popular works. 2. Longevity--Popular works. I. Title: Science and art of living a longer and healthier life. II. Schrier, Robert W. III. Title.

RA776 .B276 2000
613--dc21

                                                              99-058003

Publisher's Note
The ideas, procedures, and suggestions contained in this book are not intended as a substitute for consulting with your physician.

Printed in the United States of America

Foreword

Proust once observed that "the real voyage of discovery is not in seeking new lands but seeing with new eyes." Carl Bartecchi and Robert Schrier direct us to look at health with new eyes. Health, they suggest, is both an art and a science; and it takes an understanding of both to live a longer and healthier life. This is important both to individuals and to public policy.

A nation's health has more to do with its lifestyle and habits than with the quality of its health care system. Without casting aspersions on the brilliance of U.S. medicine (which has saved one desperately important to me), we know clearly that your best doctor is yourself. We can avoid many more diseases than we can cure. Our habits are more important than our hospitals. The authors know the most valuable thing they can do for the public is to educate people on what they can do for themselves. They recognize that "medicine" and "health" are related but are not Siamese twins.

National polls confirm that "health" is one of the American public's most important priorities. But how does one achieve a long and healthy life? The authors inform us of a wide variety of simple things we can do for ourselves. These are obvious but still too often overlooked.

Victor Fuchs has written:

> The greatest current potential for improving the health of the American people is to be found in what they do and don't do to and for themselves. Individual decisions about diet, exercise, and

smoking are of critical importance; and collective decisions affecting pollution and other aspects of the environment are also relevant.

As a public policy maker, I feel that my patient is society. It is important to distinguish between a doctor's role and a public policymaker's. Public policy must, by definition, ask macro questions, such as "How do we keep a society healthy?" and "How do we invest limited funds to buy the most health?"

I started asking these questions when I was in the Colorado legislature. I could not understand why there was (and is) an inverse correlation in the developed world between health spending and health.

The U.S., Canada, and Germany spend the most on health care; yet they have (generally) the worst health statistics. Japan spends the least and has the best. I was told that the Japanese recognized that getting people jobs and increasing living standards will buy far more health for a country than having a health care system.

The U.S. Department of Health and Human Services estimates that, of the 30 years that have been added to human life expectancy this century, only five of those years are due to clinical medicine. We all must learn better what we can do for ourselves. With all their medical training, the authors still remind us that our health depends more on ourselves than on them.

Medicine is a profession, but health policy is a public policy choice. Our government pays more than 40 percent of health care costs. Health care costs are bankrupting more and more businesses and are dampening needed wage increases. Medicare is fast heading toward bankruptcy. Our aging bodies can thus bankrupt our children. Inquiring minds increasingly ask, "How do we keep a society healthy?"

This argument is timeless. The ancient Greeks had two theories concerning health: one symbolized by the goddess Hygeia and the other by the god Aesculapius. Hygeia was the guardian of health, but her role was to symbolize the belief that people would stay in good health if they lived according to reason. She represented moderation in lifestyles, not treatment of the sick. Aesculapius, in contrast, was concerned with identifying the cause of disease and the treatment of the sick.

These divergent views of health have never been resolved and remain a key issue today, one that will grow during the next 10 years. Dr. Bartecchi and Dr. Schrier brilliantly bridge these two aspects of health. Both are scholars in allopathic medicine; yet both recognize that we currently do not inform the public enough on how people can take care of their own health. Their book is filled with useful and practical suggestions on how individuals, families, and societies can best maintain health.

The authors, thus, have risen above the excellence of their own specialties and have looked at the big picture. They are concerned with both medicine and health and have given us a practical guide to use in our daily lives.

Richard Lamm
Governor of Colorado
1975-1987

Dedication

To our wives, Kay and Barbara, who continue to help us live longer, healthier, and happier lives.

Acknowledgements

The authors wish to recognize Shirley Artese and Kay Bartecchi for expert technical assistance. We appreciate the insightful and thought-provoking quotations provided by Barbara Lindley Schrier.

About The Authors

Carl Bartecchi and Robert Schrier comprise a unique physician team that has worked together for more than a decade in several health care and educational areas. Dr. Bartecchi, a pre-eminent practitioner of internal medicine for more than 30 years, has been recognized nationally, having received both the prestigious American College of Physicians Ralph O. Claypoole Memorial Award and Colorado's Distinguished Internist Award of the American College of Physicians. Bartecchi is also Distinguished Clinical Professor of Medicine at the University of Colorado School of Medicine.

Dr. Schrier has been Professor and Chairman of the Department of Medicine at the University of Colorado for more than 23 years. He is one of the leading academicians in the world. Dr. Schrier is an Honorary Fellow of the Royal College of Physicians, a member of the Institute of Medicine of the National Academy of Sciences, and a Master of the American College of Physicians. He has authored more than 700 scientific papers and edited 40 books. Dr. Schrier has received numerous honors and awards, including the Robert H. Williams Award as the outstanding Chairman of Medicine in the country and the highest honor of the American College of Physicians, the John Phillips Memorial Award.

Although educating physicians and patients has been the continual focus of Bartecchi and Schrier, this text, *The Science and Art of Living a Longer and Healthier Life*, is written for the lay public in response to patients' requests and the need for medically sound and substantiated data. The text includes the best scientific and practical information available for individuals who desire to make reasonable efforts to extend the quality and length of their lives.

The Science and Art of Living a Longer and Healthier Life

Expert Reviewers

Richard Bakemeier, M.D., Professor of Medicine, Division of Medical Oncology, University of Colorado Health Sciences Center

Robert Ballard, M.D., Associate Professor of Medicine, Division of Pulmonary Science and Critical Care Medicine, University of Colorado Health Sciences Center

Blair Carlson, M.D., Clinical Professor of Medicine, University of Colorado Health Sciences Center

Steven Dubovsky, M.D., Professor of Psychiatry and Medicine, University of Colorado Health Sciences Center

Robert Eckel, M.D., Professor of Medicine, Division of Endocrinology, Metabolism and Diabetes, University of Colorado Health Sciences Center

William Hiatt, M.D., Professor of Medicine, Director of Colorado Prevention Center, University of Colorado Health Sciences Center

Fred Hofeldt, M.D., Professor Emeritus of Medicine, University of Colorado Health Sciences Center

Steve Johnson, M.D., Associate Professor of Medicine, Division of Infectious Diseases, University of Colorado Health Sciences Center

Stuart Linas, M.D., Professor of Medicine, Division of Renal Diseases and Hypertension, University of Colorado Health Sciences Center

Steven Mostow, M.D., Professor of Medicine, Division of Infectious Diseases, University of Colorado Health Sciences Center

Allan Prochazka, M.D., Professor of Medicine and Preventive Medicine, University of Colorado Health Sciences Center

Stuart Schneck, M.D., Professor Emeritus of Neurology, University of Colorado Health Sciences Center

Phil Wolf, M.D., Professor of Medicine, Division of Cardiology, University of Colorado Health Sciences Center

Preface

It has been almost three years since publication of the first edition of, *The Science and Art of Living a Longer and Healthier Life*. Could much have changed in three years to justify another edition? The answer is a resounding **"yes"**.

Not only have many concepts changed or been modified, but several new considerations have arrived that deserve inclusion in this new edition of our book, a book devoted to providing readers with documented strategies that can allow them to live a longer and healthier life.

At present, we are reaping the benefits from many large-scale, prospective clinical studies. These studies have provided new evidence-based insights into several difficult health problem areas. As physicians and educators, we demand proof and support for the concepts and recommendations that we pass on to our patients in order to help counter undocumented information that bombards the public via radio, television, newspapers, magazines, and Internet sources. Conflicting data that the public is asked to decipher are confusing and lessen the public's confidence in our healthcare systems. *The Science and Art of Living a Longer and Healthier Life* should resolve apparent contradictions in how to live a happy and healthier life.

We have also added a chapter on alternative medicine, in view of the present popularity of treatments generated by that discipline and its disciples. Here we ask the public to seek the same level of documentation for the premises and therapies of alternative medicine that are required of high quality, cost-effective medicine.

The Authors

Table of Contents

RISK FACTORS

DISEASE PREVENTION/HEALTH AIDS

GENERAL INFORMATION

CONCLUSION

FIGURES

TABLES

Introduction

Since the turn of the twentieth century, life expectancy of Americans has increased by about 30 years, from 45 to 75 years old. This significant gain can be attributed to various reasons, including health care, better nutrition, sanitation, occupational safety, and housing. Financially secure, industrialized nations have been able to manage many of their infectious disease problems, leaving a variety of chronic illnesses as their major health concerns. Coronary artery disease, for example, reigns as the most important cause of death and disability in the U.S. and is becoming more prevalent in less industrialized countries.

Valuable and cost-effective ways of preventing coronary artery disease are not only available but also capable of promoting general good health. One study suggests that an estimated 35 percent of the excess coronary artery disease that occurred among persons with sedentary lifestyles could have been eliminated by subjects' increasing their physical activity levels. Additionally, reducing fat intake by one to three percent reduces the overall incidence of coronary artery disease by 32,000 to 92,000 cases.

Other ways to reduce coronary artery disease are to target its leading causes, hypertension, smoking, and diabetes; other chronic illnesses can be viewed in light of their individual prevention strategies as well. Our primary goal should be to prevent the appearance of disease in those with no signs or symptoms, but achieving this goal often involves efforts that must be initiated early in life, e.g., promoting healthy habits in children.

Certainly accidents, wars, natural disasters, and the unfortunate acquisition of certain diseases can abruptly terminate life, but it has been estimated that 50 percent of premature deaths are associated with choices people make, including abuse of tobacco, alcohol, and other toxic substances; unhealthy diets; and sedentary lifestyles. Further significant reductions in premature deaths can be accomplished by reducing environmental risks and improving access to medical treatment.

Today more than ever, scientific studies and observations indicate that almost anyone's lifespan, from almost any age as a starting point, can be extended by incorporating certain reasonable, rational, and inexpensive actions or strategies into the lifestyle. Unfortunately, there is no guarantee regarding quality of the extended period of life, but it appears that these same principles often also contribute to improved quality of extended life. Accomplishing life extension requires positive actions and definite commitments by those interested in such a long-term goal.

This discussion is directed to individuals in their mid-20s and beyond. Younger individuals tend to be preoccupied by other, more pressing concerns as well as protected by a certain feeling of immortality. Though without proof, the authors' personal feelings are that the 40th birthday appears to trigger early thoughts of "just how long the ol' bod can make it" for most people.

We all arrive in this world with a genetic makeup that has an important influence on the quality and length of our lives. In the future, genetic engineering can be expected to help improve chances for a better and a longer life. For now, though, the tried and tested actions and principles that are supported by studies in the medical literature and reinforced by successful trials of large numbers of individuals are the standards to be used. The authors have taken care to avoid unreasonable or overly expensive recommendations that would not be available to the general public or that would serve to advertise or endorse products touted as capable of extending life.

The subjects of the following chapters are associated with principles or actions that have the potential to prolong life. First, however, is a look at the causes of death from different viewpoints, those of the National Foundation for Infectious Diseases and of the National Center for Health Statistics.

From the National Foundation for Infectious Diseases, 1996-97 Injury Chartbook, Hyattsville, Maryland, 1997, leading causes of death in the U.S. in 1995 were:

CAUSE	NUMBER OF DEATHS
1. Heart disease	737,563
2. Cancer	538,455
3. Cerebrovascular disease	157,991
4. Chronic obstructive pulmonary disease	102,899
5. Unintentional injury	93,320
6. Pneumonia and influenza	82,923
7. Diabetes	59,254
8. HIV and AIDS	43,115
9. Suicide	31,284
10. Chronic liver diseases	25,222

From McGinnis and Foege, who point out that, of the approximately 2.14 million U.S residents who died in 1990, approximately half died of particular preventable causes, leading causes of death were:

CAUSE	NUMBER OF DEATHS	PERCENTAGE OF TOTAL DEATHS
1. Tobacco	400,000	19
2. Dietary factors and activity patterns	300,000	14
3. Alcohol	100,000	5
4. Microbial agents	90,000	4
5. Toxic agents	60,000	3
6. Firearms	35,000	2
7. High risk sexual behavior	30,000	1
8. Motor vehicle injuries	25,000	1
9. Illicit use of drugs	20,000	< 1
Total	**1,060,000**	**49**

Further Reading

McGinnis JM, Foege WH: Actual causes of death in the United States. JAMA 1993;270.

Coronary Artery Disease: The Major Cause of Death in the U.S.

Avoid fried foods, which angry up the blood. If your stomach disputes you, lie down and pacify it with cool thoughts. Keep the juices flowing by jangling around gently as you move. Go very light on the vices, such as carrying on in society. The social ramble ain't restful. Don't look back. Something might be gaining on you.

-Satchel Paige

Facts

1. Coronary artery disease accounts for more than one-half of cardiovascular deaths and about one-third of all deaths in the U.S.

2. Heart attack is the single largest killer of American males and females.

3. This year as many as 1,500,000 Americans will have new or recurrent heart attacks and about one-third of these people will die.

4. Twenty-seven percent of men and 44 percent of women die within one year of having a heart attack.

5. Persons known to be at high risk for coronary disease die 10 to 15 years earlier if they smoke.

6. It is estimated that passive smoking causes almost 40,000 heart disease deaths yearly in the U.S.

7. Men who consume high-fiber diets (especially fiber from grains) have significantly lower risks of heart attack than those whose diets are poor in fiber-rich foods.

8. In patients with adult-onset (Type 2, noninsulin-dependent) diabetes mellitus, death from coronary disease is increased 200 percent in males and 400 percent in females.

9. Physical inactivity is associated with at least a twofold increase in risk for coronary artery disease events.

10. Up to 80 percent of people who develop heart disease could have been identified and treated years earlier if their risk factors had been known.

11. Seventy percent of heart attacks occur in patients with coronary arteries less than 50-percent occluded.

Coronary artery disease is the leading cause of death for both men and women, accounting for almost 500,000 deaths in the U.S. each year. Since 1970, however, the death rate for coronary artery disease has declined almost 50 percent due to factors relating to treatment of major risk factors.

Atherosclerosis results in blockages or hardening of coronary arteries with formation of plaque. The resultant obstruction of blood flow through the arteries causes heart attacks, heart rhythm disturbances, heart failure, and/or the numerous complications known to be associated with heart attacks. In recent years, it has become apparent that there are cardiovascular risk factors that predispose individuals to developing atherosclerosis and its subsequent complications and, thus, increase these individuals' risks for coronary artery disease. Though it is possible for people to have heart attacks and die despite having no risk factors, it is clearly documented that individuals with greater numbers of risk factors, and especially those with recognized problematic risk factors, have the greatest danger of developing coronary disease. Surveys of large groups suggest that less than 20 percent of such groups are free of all commonly recognized risk factors. However, there are many potential candidates that someday may prove valuable as new risk factors for coronary artery disease.

Risk factors can be viewed in several ways. Some cannot be changed; these include:
○ Age
○ Sex
○ Race
○ Heredity

Other risk factors lend themselves to change and have different degrees of importance, the most serious being:

- Hypertension
- Cigarette smoking
- High cholesterol levels
- Diabetes mellitus
- Enlarged heart
- Cocaine use
- Homocysteine

Actions that effectively modify these risk factors include:

- Dietary control
- Use of medications
- Quitting smoking
- Exercise
- Diabetes control
- Avoiding cocaine use

Other important modifiable risk factors include:

- Obesity
- Menopause
- Sedentary lifestyle
- Excessive alcohol consumption
- Oral contraceptive use
- Stress
- Setting at the time of a first heart attack, e.g.:
  - An individual living alone
  - A recent spousal loss or separation
  - Evidence of lack of social support
- Factors involved with blood clotting:
  - Platelets
  - Fibrinogen
  - Factor VII

Corrective actions can effectively modify risk factors. Protective actions include:

- Use of estrogen in menopausal women
- Increased exercise
- Moderate alcohol consumption (one to two glasses of wine per day)
- Enhanced HDL (good) cholesterol
- Use of aspirin

Cigarette smoking is the most dangerous risk factor for coronary artery disease. Quitting smoking allows the risk for coronary artery disease to revert to that of a nonsmoker within two to three years.

While cholesterol levels are important, it should be recognized that about half of people with coronary artery disease have normal cholesterol profiles. Some in that group, however, will also be found to have high triglyceride and low HDL cholesterol levels, a bad combination that has been shown to be associated with increased risk for coronary artery disease.

With regard to hypertension, both systolic and diastolic pressures are important and must be controlled to reduce the incidence of heart attack and stroke.

Numerous studies have shown that regular exercise can help prevent a first heart attack. Such exercise can be associated with a number of desirable goals, including:

- Maintaining desirable body weight
- Elevating HDL (good) cholesterol
- Improving work capacity of the heart
- Reducing blood pressure
- Helping to manage stress

Commonly seen combinations of the most important risk factors (e.g., hypertension plus cigarette smoking plus high cholesterol) can be particularly lethal. Another bad combination is the use of oral contraceptives in women who smoke. Correcting modifiable risk factors can prevent much morbidity and mortality. The earlier that persons with modifiable risk factors are aware of and change these risk factors, the greater the chance of avoiding their otherwise lethal consequences. Modifying major risk factors, such as smoking, high blood pressure, and high cholesterol levels, definitely reduces the risk of heart attack and its resulting complications. Risk factor modification, especially for patients with known coronary artery disease, improves survival rates.

Other interesting but often complex risk factors are important but are discussed here only briefly. These include elevated lipoprotein (a) levels, elevated fasting insulin levels in nondiabetics, and substantial amounts of small, dense LDL particles. Lipoprotein (a), especially at high blood levels, appears to be able to encourage the formation of blood clots. Also, like LDL, which it resembles, lipoprotein (a), can be deposited in the walls of arteries. Increased blood levels of insulin also appear to be associated with greater risk of clot formation in coronary arteries that are already compromised. The size and density of LDL particles can be important factors in estimating coronary artery disease risk. Patients with small, dense particles have three times the risk of coronary artery disease as those with large LDL particles.

Recommendations

1. Assess, with the help of a physician, your cardiovascular risk factor status and reevaluate it regularly.
2. If you smoke, STOP.
3. Eat a heart-healthy diet, specifically a diet with less fat, less meat, and more fiber-rich foods such as fresh fruits and vegetables. Eat at least five portions of fruits and vegetables daily.
4. Maintain normal blood pressure levels, i.e., 140/ 90 mm Hg or lower (except for diabetics, who should maintain levels of 130/85 mm Hg or lower).
5. Exercise regularly, i.e., 30 minutes per day seven days per week.
6. If you are overweight, reduce and aim for desirable weight.
7. Use alcohol only in moderation, i.e., one to two glasses of wine per day for males and one glass per day for females.
8. Postmenopausal women can benefit from estrogen replacement unless contraindications exist.
9. Never use cocaine. Even the first use of this drug can be lethal or lead to permanent cardiac damage.
10. If you are a male age 50 years or older and have multiple cardiovascular risk factors, taking aspirin at 81 to 325 mg per day may be of value unless contraindications exist. Contraindications include poorly controlled hypertension, ulcers, and bleeding problems.
11. If you are an adult-onset, Type 2 diabetic, weight loss may actually "cure" your diabetes or at least allow for better blood sugar control. A five-percent weight loss maintained over two years has been shown to prevent adult diabetes in high-risk, middle-aged individuals.

12. Carefully review Chapters 2 (high blood pressure), 5 (diabetes), 12 (smoking), 13 (cholesterol), 14 (obesity), 18 (diet), and 19 (exercise) of this book and follow the recommendations provided in each.

Further Reading

Twenty-seventh Bethesda Conference. Matching the Intensity of Risk Factor Management with the Hazard for Coronary Disease Events. J Am Col Cardiol, April 1996.

Heart and Stroke Facts: 1996 Statistical Supplement. American Heart Association.

High Blood Pressure: The Silent Killer

To be 70 years young is sometimes far more cheerful and hopeful than to be 40 years old.

-Oliver Wendell Holmes

Facts

1. More than half of all Americans older than age 65 have high blood pressure.

2. For patients ages 60 or older, treatment of high blood pressure can reduce mortality from all causes by 12 percent, from stroke by 36 percent, and from coronary artery disease by 25 percent.

3. Studies suggest that reducing diastolic blood pressure by five to six points in all hypertensives may lower the incidence of coronary artery disease by 14 percent and stroke by 42 percent.

4. Only 24 percent of hypertensive individuals are thought to have their blood pressure levels under optimal control.

5. Statistics show that only 65 percent of individuals with blood pressure levels at or above 140/90 mm Hg were informed of their elevated blood pressures.

6. Numerous factors can distort blood pressure readings, including location (doctor's office), instrument error, blood pressure cuff size, recent exertion, and observer error (hearing problems).

7. Many prescribed medications can cause high blood pressure.

8. In 1993, high blood pressure killed 37,520 Americans and contributed to the deaths of thousands more.

Hypertension is a common, important, and very controllable cause of stroke, heart failure, and coronary artery disease, especially in the elderly. Hypertension accelerates hardening of the arteries and is, thus, one of the leading risk factors for heart attack and stroke. Large numbers of people die from the heart attacks, strokes, and kidney failure caused by hypertension.

Hypertension, termed the "silent killer", is usually a symptomless disease, often discovered during routine health evaluations or screenings. Studies have shown that more than 30 percent of patients are unaware of their disease. Of those who are aware, only about one-half are under treatment; and of these, only about one-quarter are well controlled.

It is now recognized that, as blood pressure levels rise above 110/80 mm Hg, the risk of cardiovascular disease increases. Repeated blood pressures at or above 140/90 mm Hg fall in the hypertension range. It should be noted that blood pressure readings taken in the doctor's office are higher than those taken away from the office in about 80 percent of cases. Previously, the diastolic pressure (lower number) was considered the more important; but more recently it has been recognized that the systolic pressure, which reflects blood pressure in the arteries when the heart contracts, is more important for estimating risks of stroke and heart attack. Often systolic hypertension only is found in elderly patients.

In persons with high cardiovascular risks (i.e., those with diabetes, heart failure, or kidney failure), the blood pressure goal should be 130/85 mm Hg or lower. Diabetic patients especially appear to benefit from a diastolic blood pressure of 80 mm Hg or lower. Such levels can be accomplished initially through lifestyle changes and, if needed later, drug therapies.

Controlling hypertension may not require the use of medications, however. To some degree, lifestyle modifications can be effective in all patients; modifications may include:

○ Weight reduction
○ Moderate alcohol intake
○ Reduced sodium (salt) intake
○ Regular physical activity
○ Smoking cessation

Alcohol use can cause hypertension and is a reversible cause of high blood pressure. It is estimated that, in about eight percent of American men with hypertension, the cause is excessive alcohol use.

Recently, a diet that was low in fat and high in fruits, vegetables, low-fat dairy products, and whole grains was found to lower blood pressure levels effectively. Adequate potassium intake from fruits and vegetables, nonfat dairy products, or supplements also appears to be important for blood pressure control. Although potassium has the ability to lower blood pressure, supplements must be taken with caution to avoid excess supplies. Salt restriction, important for all hypertension patients, is especially important in Blacks, who tend to be sensitive to salt.

Blood pressure levels not controlled by these measures must be treated with drugs that have proven to be effective, especially in the elderly. For this population, drug therapy has reduced the incidence of stroke by one-third and heart attack by one-fourth. Deaths have been reduced by at least 10 percent for drug therapy patients.

Patients with hypertension must work closely with their physicians for the best results. They should have home blood pressure monitors to keep track of their own progress. Advantages of home blood pressure measurements are many, including:

- Blood pressures taken on physicians' office monitors tend to be higher than those taken on home monitors
- Medications added for control of blood pressure can be monitored more closely
- Concerns about symptoms related to high and low blood pressure levels can be resolved quickly
- Stresses, activities, and/or other illnesses that affect blood pressure can be detected quickly and adjustments in therapy employed rapidly

Patients should inform their physicians about other medications they are taking that are known to elevate blood pressure. These include:

- Female hormones
- Certain arthritis medications
- Cold remedies
- Appetite suppressants
- Cocaine
- Certain antidepressant medications
- Anabolic steroids (used for muscle building)

Nonsteroidal anti-inflammatory drugs (NSAIDs), those used to treat aches, pains, and arthritis, are popular in the U.S. These drugs, however, can elevate blood pressure in some people, especially the elderly and those with hypertension or kidney problems, and can also blunt the effects of some antihypertensive medications. Some NSAIDs are more likely to cause problems than others; aspirin and sulindac (Clinoril®), for example, are less likely to affect blood pressure than some others. Adverse effects of more harmful over-the-counter drugs may not be recognized and can lead to problems.

Advantages of treating hypertension can be seen within months of initiating therapy and can occur even if blood pressure levels are not lowered to the most desirable range.

Drugs used to treat hypertension can have major and at times life-threatening complications, especially in the elderly in whom age-related changes affect the way drugs are used, altered, and/or eliminated from their bodies. Patients must discuss with their physicians any significant changes they detect after starting, changing, or modifying medication programs.

A recent study suggests that taking one baby aspirin (81 mg) per day is valuable and safe for hypertension patients and may reduce the incidence of major cardiovascular problems by 15 percent and heart attack by 36 percent; no effect has been noted for stroke rates.

Recommendations

1. Even if blood pressure measurements are normal, you should have your blood pressure checked at least every two years.

2. Work closely with your physician to achieve good blood pressure control.

3. Be able to take your own blood pressure.

4. Understand your blood pressure medications. Ask your physician or pharmacist for written information about each drug. Patient-oriented information about drugs can be obtained easily.

5. NEVER stop taking blood pressure medications on your own. Stopping certain medications can result in especially severe blood pressure elevations with major complications (stroke, heart failure, or heart attack). A common cause of poor blood pressure control is patients not taking their medications because of side effects or costs.

6. Avoid nondrug or natural treatments that, though often unproven, commonly are recommended for treating hypertension. These therapies, which include biofeedback, yoga, meditation, acupuncture, hypnosis, and certain fad diets, are not of the same proven effectiveness as other standard therapies and, thus, are of questionable value for effective, long-term blood pressure control.

7. The most important nonmedication treatments for hypertension are smoking cessation, weight loss, salt restriction, and exercise. Among these, smoking cessation is the most important; cardiovascular complications are increased several-fold in hypertensive patients who smoke. Weight loss of as little as five to 10 percent may control blood pressure with fewer and/or lower doses of antihypertensive medications.

Approximately 20 percent of hypertension patients have increased blood pressure levels when ingesting large amounts of salt (i.e., French fries, chips, etc.). Thus, moderate salt restriction, achieved by avoiding canned goods and salty foods and by not salting foods, may help blood pressure control. This is especially true of African-Americans, the elderly, and diabetic patients whose blood pressures are "salt-sensitive". While exercise does not appear to decrease blood pressure as much as weight loss, it does lower the increased cardiovascular risk that is common in the hypertension patient.

8. As high blood pressure and high cholesterol are additive with respect to cardiovascular complications, high cholesterol must be treated more aggressively in hypertension patients than normotensive patients.

Stroke:
How to Prevent the Third Most Common Cause of Death in the U.S.

Do what you can with what you have, where you are.

-Theodore Roosevelt

Facts

1. Stroke is the second most common cause of death worldwide.

2. Stroke is the third leading cause of death, after heart disease and cancer, in the U.S.

3. Each year about 550,000 Americans suffer new or recurrent strokes.

4. The incidence of stroke more than doubles each decade after age 55.

5. High blood pressure is a major contributing factor in up to 70 percent of strokes.

6. The patient who survives an initial stroke has a recurrence rate of up to 18 percent during the following year. About 31 percent of stroke victims die within a year.

7. Stroke is the leading cause of serious long-term disability in the U.S.

8. Smokers have significantly greater risks for stroke than nonsmokers.

9. A smoker with high blood pressure has 20 times the risk of stroke as a nonsmoker with normal blood pressure.

Stroke is the third leading cause of death and the leading cause of serious disability in the U.S. Each year, half a million people, about 12 of every 10,000 Americans, suffer strokes, and about 150,000 people die from them. The risk of having a stroke increases with age, the risk being highest after age 55. The risk is higher in men until the mid-50s, when it begins to equal that of women. The risk of having a stroke also increases with family history (i.e., a close relative who has had a stroke, heart attack, or transient ischemic attack [TIA]).

New therapies to reduce the severity of stroke are under study, but these must be administered within three hours of onset of a stroke. Strokes can be prevented by identifying and treating people at high risk before the problem develops and by controlling risk factors. Controllable risk factors for stroke include:

- High blood pressure - Hypertension (systolic pressure greater than 140 mm Hg and diastolic pressure greater than 90 mm Hg) may be the cause of 40 percent of strokes. Improved treatment of high blood pressure over the past 25 years has been credited with the major reduction in stroke mortality during that period. Many studies have shown that lowering systolic blood pressure and maintaining good blood pressure control by almost any antihypertensive medication, has been effective in preventing stroke. Both systolic and diastolic hypertension needs to be treated and controlled.
- Cigarette smoking - Smokers are 50 percent more likely to have strokes than nonsmokers; cigarette smoking predisposes to stroke by a variety of defined mechanisms. Those who quit smoking have about the same risk of stroke as nonsmokers.

- Diabetes - It is estimated that diabetes can double the risk of stroke. The mechanism for this is not completely clear, but diabetes is a risk factor for cerebral arteriosclerosis. Contrary to the expected, improving blood sugar control in insulin-dependent diabetics does not appear to reduce the incidence of stroke. Strokes that occur in the setting of high levels of blood sugar, however, tend to be more severe and disabling. Controlling blood pressure has been shown to decrease the occurrence of stroke in adult diabetic patients.

- Heart disease - Heart rhythm disturbances (e.g., atrial fibrillation, heart failure, heart attack, previous heart valve disease, or heart valve replacement) can increase the likelihood of stroke. Atrial fibrillation, a common cause of irregular heart rhythm in the elderly, can increase risks of stroke to as high as seven percent each year. Medications, including blood thinners, and surgery can significantly reduce stroke risks in these patients.

- Vascular disease - Significant blockage of the carotid artery in the neck (greater than 70 percent narrowing) occurs in about five percent of the elderly. Even if these patients are without symptoms, stroke risks are three to four percent each year. This disorder can be managed by medications, with or without surgery. However, depending on associated factors, as many as five percent of patients who elect surgery may suffer a stroke or die from the procedure itself. The physician will listen to the area over the carotid artery in the neck with a stethoscope to find evidence of blockage in the carotid artery. If found, further testing will determine the degree of blockage.

- Transient ischemic attacks (TIAs) - The risk of stroke is increased in those who have had TIAs. Up to 20 percent of these people will subsequently have a stroke. Aspirin and other medications have been shown to reduce the risk of stroke in patients with TIAs, which are evidenced by fleeting or transient episodes of:
  - Unilateral weakness
  - Numbness
  - Distortion of speech
  - Loss of vision
  - Unsteadiness
  - Double vision
- Cholesterol – Elevated cholesterol levels, alone or accompanied by other cardiovascular risk factors, contribute to the development of atherosclerosis in the arteries that supply the brain. Many studies have shown that cholesterol-lowering drugs (statins) are capable of significantly reducing risks of stroke in people with lipid problems, especially those with coronary artery disease. Eating diets such as the Mediterranean diet (low saturated fat, high monounsaturated fat, lots of fruits and vegetables) is also valuable. A recent study from Harvard, reported that people who ate up to six servings of fruits and vegetables daily were at more than a 30 percent lower risk of having a stroke compared with people who ate less than three servings daily.
- Alcohol - Moderate alcohol intake (not more than two drinks daily) may be associated with a protective effect against stroke; however, heavy alcohol intake, especially in men and in those with hypertension, has been associated with an increased risk of stroke.

◉ Oral contraceptive use – Women who take oral contraceptives have an increased risk of stroke. This is especially a problem for women older than age 35, for women who smoke, and for women who take older, higher-dose hormone pills.

Though many believe that type A behavior, depression, hopelessness, anxiety, psychological stress, and highly emotional life events could be risk factors for stroke, existing data do not support this possibility.

There is some suggestion that unrecognized or "silent" strokes occur in the elderly and are manifest only by a significant decline in intellectual ability. Older individuals appear also to be at greater risk of developing the more commonly recognized stroke picture.

Besides medications and surgical treatment, other approaches to avoiding stroke are recommended. These methods act by preventing or limiting further vascular lesions, controlling blood pressure, or providing nutrients or antioxidants that may prove helpful. This approach involves the maintenance of a low-cholesterol, low-fat diet with plenty of fruits, vegetables, and grains at a calorie level sufficient to maintain healthy weight. Also valuable are daily exercise and the avoidance of salt, if patients have tendencies to high blood pressure.

For those with arterial disease that cause ischemic (deficient blood supply) events such as TIAs, aspirin is the drug of first choice for stroke prevention. Aspirin reduces the relative risk of stroke by about 25 percent, with minimal side effects. The best dose of aspirin for stroke prevention has not been determined, but doses ranging from those in a baby aspirin to two regular aspirins daily are effective. For those who cannot tolerate aspirin, clopidogrel (Plavix®) is the drug of second choice.

Up to 85 percent of strokes that occur in the U.S. each year are ischemic strokes, with the remainder of the hemorrhagic variety. A new approach to treating acute ischemic stroke is the "clot-buster", a tissue plasminogen activator (TPA) that, when given within three hours of the onset of stroke symptoms, has proved to be quite effective, with patients 30-percent more likely to have minimal or no disabilities three months after such treatment compared to those not receiving this agent. Unfortunately, only about five percent of acute stroke patients receive this therapy because of their inability to reach hospital emergency rooms within the three-hour period. Strokes, like heart attacks, are medical emergencies. People must become familiar with stroke symptoms (see TIAs) and seek help immediately if treatments such as this are to be effective. Once in the emergency room, patients should be studied to determine and, if possible, eliminate cerebral hemorrhage and other problems that can contraindicate clot-buster therapy.

Patients with acute ischemic stroke who are not eligible for clot-busting therapy should be started on aspirin at 160 to 325 mg per day within 48 hours of initial stroke symptoms. Aspirin also is valuable for its ability to prevent recurrent stroke in those who have already had a stroke.

Other factors that are also important in preventing an initial or subsequent stroke include exercising, avoiding illicit drug use (cocaine, amphetamines), and controlling weight. Individuals with blood clotting abnormalities and homocysteine problems will benefit from correcting these factors as they can. It is not known, however, if the easily reduced homocysteine levels will lower incidences of cardiovascular disease and stroke. It appears prudent, though, to control homocysteine levels by ensuring adequate levels of folate and vitamins B_6 and B_{12} in the body through adequate intakes of vegetables, fruits, legumes, meat, fish, and fortified grains and cereals. In specific cases in which intake of certain food supplies cannot be accomplished, simple multivitamin preparations should prove useful in providing the necessary folate and B vitamins. There is also some evidence that diets rich in potassium (high levels of fruits and vegetables) can reduce risks of stroke.

Recommendations

1. Recognize that acute stroke is a medical emergency that should be evaluated in a hospital emergency room as quickly as possible.
2. Do not smoke.
3. Know your blood pressure level and check it often as you age.
4. Eat at least five servings of fresh fruits and vegetables daily.
5. Be able to recognize warning signs of TIAs.
6. Notify your physician if your heart beats irregularly.
7. Exercise daily and aim for an ideal weight.

Cancer on the Rise:
How to Screen for Early Detection
and Treatment

That which does not kill me makes me stronger.

-Nietzsche

Facts

1. Thirty percent of all cancers are caused by tobacco.

2. Smoking and diet may cause up to two-thirds of U.S. cancer deaths.

3. Diet, particularly high-fat and low-fiber, is a significant factor in cancer deaths in the U.S.

4. Individuals who are 40 percent over ideal weight have as high as a 55-percent greater risk of dying from cancer than those of normal weight.

5. Lung cancer is the leading cause of cancer-related deaths in both males and females in the U.S.

6. Man-made chemicals, artificial sweeteners, pesticides, and food additives are relatively insignificant or minor causes of cancer.

7. About 60 percent of human lung cancers contain mutations in the P53 tumor suppressor gene. A recent study shows a direct link between a defined cigarette smoke carcinogen (benzo [a] pyrene) and human cancer mutations.

Cancer is the leading cause of morbidity and mortality in the U.S.; and if current trends continue, it will soon become the leading cause of death. Presently more than 500,000 Americans die from cancer each year.

One-third of all Americans will eventually contract cancer. An increase in the number of cases of cancer has been recognized, but some of this is related to our population growth.

The significant growth in the number of older adults is another important factor. It has been estimated that more than 60 percent of all cancers occur after age 60 and 36 percent after age 70.

Cancer, of course, is not a single disease. There are many different forms of cancer, each with their own patterns of progression and potentials for early detection, treatment, and prognosis. A relatively small number of cancers make up the majority of cancer cases; these are:

Males	Females
Lung	Lung
Colorectal	Breast
Prostate	Colorectal
Bladder	Ovarian
Lymphoma	Uterine

Of these cancers, lung, breast, prostate, and colorectal account for more than 50 percent of all cancer deaths. Some tumors are more prevalent than might be suspected. Studies of the prostate gland during autopsy, for example, indicate that unsuspected tumors occur in 30 percent of males at age 50 and as many as 100 percent of males by age 90.

Cancers can develop from any combination of genetic, chemical, physical, or biologic insults to a body's cells. Involved is usually a complex interplay of genetics, diet, lifestyle, and environmental factors.

Because effective treatments for many cancers are not always available, the best method appears to be prevention and/or early detection. The National Cancer Institute has estimated that early detection practices could reduce U.S. cancer mortality rates by 25 percent. Early detection is useful for cancers of the:

- Breast
- Uterine cervix
- Skin
- Mouth
- Thyroid
- Colon
- Endometrium
- Prostate
- Testicle
- Urinary bladder

Efforts to prevent cancers are useful for cancers of the:

- Lung
- Head and neck
- Skin
- Breast
- Colon
- Cervix

The opportunity to prevent cancers becomes apparent after considering that:

⊙ About 90 percent of lung cancers among men and 79 percent among women (87 percent overall) are due to cigarette smoking.

⊙ Ninety percent of skin cancers could be prevented by protection from the sun's rays.

⊙ Seventeen thousand cancer deaths each year are related to excessive alcohol use. These are primarily cancers of the mouth and upper gastrointestinal tract (i.e., esophagus and stomach) and are more likely to occur in persons who both smoke and have excessive alcohol intake. One large study suggests that breast cancer increases by 30 percent in women who consume three to six drinks per week and by 60 percent in women who consumed more than nine drinks per week.

⊙ Eating a healthful diet may prevent as many as one-third of all cancer deaths. The National Cancer Institute estimates that 30,000 lives in the U.S. could be saved in the year 2000 if dietary habits were modified, particularly by eating high-fiber, low-fat diets as found with increased fresh fruit and vegetable intakes.

⊙ Individuals 40 percent or more overweight increase their risks of cancers of the:
  ⊙ Colon
  ⊙ Breast
  ⊙ Prostate
  ⊙ Gallbladder
  ⊙ Ovary
  ⊙ Uterus

- Epidemiological studies have shown that daily consumption of fresh fruits and vegetables is associated with decreased risks of cancers of the:
  - Lung
  - Prostate
  - Bladder
  - Esophagus
  - Colon/rectum
  - Stomach
  - Cervix
- Eating a high-fiber diet appears to reduce the risk of colon cancer.
- Eating a high-fat diet may be a factor in the development of cancers of the:
  - Breast
  - Colon
  - Prostate
- People who consume diets high in salt-cured and smoked foods have higher incidences of cancers of the:
  - Esophagus
  - Stomach
- Estrogen therapy in some women can increase the risk of endometrial cancer and possibly breast cancer; however, the benefits in preventing osteoporosis and heart disease are considered to outweigh the small increased risk of cancer.
- Increased risks of cancers can occur from exposure to:
  - Certain tumor-killing drugs
  - Industrial agents (asbestos) and pollutants
  - Radiation
  - Gases (radon)

Women, including those up to their early 50s, who do aerobic exercises (e.g., running, biking, walking) for four hours or more each week appear less likely to develop breast cancer.

Eating large amounts of red meat (lamb, beef, or pork) or processed meat (sausages, canned meat, hamburgers, and meats that are *smoked*, *salted*, or *cured* [e.g., bacon]) is associated with a higher risk of colorectal cancer. Meats that are prepared by grilling (i.e., broiling), barbecuing, roasting, or frying develop toxic materials on their surfaces, which in some individuals might be associated with polyp formation and bowel cancer.

In one study of stomach cancer, those who ate beef medium well or well done had more than three times the risk of developing stomach cancer than those who ate meat rare or medium rare, a result that suggests a relationship of some cancers to cooking habits. Also of interest is the fact that gravy made from meat drippings contains large amounts of cancer causing agents. High consumption of meat is also associated with prostate and pancreatic cancers. The *safest ways of cooking* meat are by baking, stewing, and boiling.

Vitamin supplements have not been proven to prevent any cancers and could in fact be harmful (see Chapter 21).

Although it is known that diets rich in fruits and vegetables lower risks of developing many types of cancers, the exact agent in these foods that lowers cancer risks is not known. Numerous studies have shown that foods high in vitamins C and E, beta-carotene, and other antioxidants are associated with lower risks for virtually all cancers; but specific vitamin supplements themselves have not proven effective and may potentially prove harmful. It appears that it is the actual, natural food product itself and not the antioxidant supplement that provides the protective benefit. Plant foods are loaded with bioactive substances in various mixtures and in combinations with minerals, little-studied chemicals, and numerous unknown contributors that, in some ill-defined way, protect us from many cancers. What we need to do for beneficial effects is to eat a minimum of five servings of a variety of fruits and vegetables each day.

New studies in the dietary areas continue to bring forth useful information. For example, lycopene, a plant chemical that gives tomatoes their red color, alone or possibly with other substances in tomatoes appears to reduce risks of developing prostate cancer. The study that showed this benefit used 10 servings (one serving was equal to one medium tomato, one-half cup of tomato or spaghetti sauce, or one-fourth cup of tomato paste) per week of cooked tomato products.

Another recent study surprisingly suggested that a high-fiber diet did not appear to be linked to decreased risks of colon cancer. The American Cancer Society, however, holds to its belief that, of the many scientific studies on the subject, the great majority do show that eating fruits and vegetables (especially green and dark yellow vegetables and those in the cabbage family), soy products, and legumes has a protective effect.

The American Cancer Society also offers guidelines for early cancer detection in people without symptoms. It recommends cancer-related check-ups by physicians every three years for persons ages 20 to 39 and annually for those ages 40 and older. Individuals at particular risks for certain cancers or with strong family histories, however, should be

evaluated more frequently. The American Cancer Society recommends that check-ups include:
- Health counseling (e.g., how to quit smoking)
- Exams for cancers of the:
  - Breast
  - Uterus
  - Cervix
  - Colon
  - Rectum
  - Prostate
  - Mouth
  - Skin
  - Testes
  - Thyroid
  - Lymph nodes

That such screening is valuable is apparent, especially in the case of breast cancer. Studies suggest that, if all women ages 50 to 69 underwent appropriate examinations along with mammography annually, their mortality rate would decline 30 to 40 percent.

To maintain the proper perspective, it is re-emphasized that smoking and improper diets are the causes of approximately two-thirds of U.S. cancer deaths, about 25 to 40 percent and 30 percent, respectively.

Recommendations (Modified from the American Cancer Society)

FOR CANCER PREVENTION
1. Stop smoking, do not use smokeless tobacco, and avoid second-hand smoke.
2. Maintain a desirable weight.
3. Eat a varied diet with lots of high-fiber foods, such as whole grain cereal, breads, and pastas.

4. Eat fruits and vegetables, at least five servings daily.
5. Cut down on total fat intake (less than 30 percent of total caloric intake).
6. Limit alcohol consumption to no more than two drinks daily.
7. Limit consumption of salt-cured, smoked, and nitrate-cured foods.
8. Keep sun exposure to a minimum; use appropriate sunscreens.
9. Discuss needs vs risks of estrogen and progesterone replacement with your doctor.
10. Recognize and avoid occupational cancer hazards and potential radiation problems.
11. Avoid all unproven herbal supplements for prevention or treatment of cancers.

FOR BREAST CANCER SCREENING
1. Women ages 20 and older should do monthly breast self-examinations.
2. Women ages 40 to 49 should have mammograms every one to two years, at the physician's discretion, and clinical breast examinations every year. The American Cancer Society, however, recently recommended once yearly mammograms for all women in their 40s.
3. Women ages 50 to 69 should have annual clinical breast examinations and mammograms. A review of screening effectiveness studies has led to the conclusion that such screening can reduce breast cancer mortality by 20 to 30 percent.
4. For women ages 70 and older, evidence of benefit is limited and conflicting. Physicians' recommendations should be heeded.

FOR CERVICAL CANCER SCREENING

Women ages 18 and older and those who were sexually active at younger ages should have Pap tests and pelvic examinations at least every three years and possibly yearly according to some recommendations. Performing Pap tests every three years reduces invasive cervical cancer rates by 91.2 percent. Only a slightly greater reduction of 93.3 percent results from annual screening. Regular testing can probably terminate at age 65 for women who have had regular previous screening with normal Pap smears. Worldwide studies show that mortality from cervical cancer has been reduced by 20 to 60 percent since the implementation of cervical cancer screening programs.

FOR COLORECTAL CANCER SCREENING

Screening for colorectal cancer is recommended for all persons ages 50 and older. Annual fecal occult blood tests and sigmoidoscopy screening every three to five years currently appears reasonable. Every five to 10 years, a barium enema may be performed in place of the sigmoidoscopy; and every 10 years, a colonoscopy may be performed in place of the sigmoidoscopy or barium enema. A one-time colonoscopy appears to be a reasonable screening approach for individuals older than age 60.

Monitoring a high-risk patient requires a colonoscopy at least every three years. A colonoscopy, with the removal of all colonic adenomas, lowers the risk of colorectal cancer by 76 to 90 percent. Studies have documented a 31- to 57-percent reduction in colon cancer risk among persons who receive fecal occult blood testing. Earlier screening should be done for those with family histories or prior diagnoses of familial polyposis or ulcerative colitis.

FOR PROSTATE CANCER SCREENING

Digital rectal examination alone will miss 30 to 40 percent of prostate cancers. The best method for early detection of prostate cancer is to combine the digital rectal exam with measurement of the prostate-specific antigen (PSA). Not everyone agrees that regular PSA testing is important; however, the American Urologic Association and American Cancer Society recommend annual screening for men ages 50 and older and earlier for Black men or men with family histories of the disease. Men with life expectancies of less than 10 years should not be screened. The PSA test does not always indicate the presence or absence of prostate cancer; in fact, only 20 to 35 percent of men with elevated PSAs have prostate cancer. A slightly elevated PSA might indicate only prostate enlargement, which is common as men age, or prostate inflammation. Up to 20 percent of localized and curable prostate cancers can be associated with a normal PSA but are detected by a rectal examination.

PSA Levels and Prostate Cancer (in percent)	
PSA Level	**Probability of Prostate cancer**
4 to 10	20 to 50 percent
Above 10	50 to 75 percent
Above 20	90 percent

One definite value of PSA screening is its ability to detect prostate cancer in young men, in which the disease is often more aggressive. PSA screening should lead to further studies and an array of available treatments, all with their own potential risks and benefits that physicians must study and explain to their patients.

FOR OTHER CANCER SCREENINGS

As part of the periodic examination, physicians should examine for cancers of the:

- Skin
- Mouth
- Testes

It is helpful for patients to point out to their physicians new, suspicious, or changing lesions on any parts of their bodies.

Diabetes:
Learning More About
Management

If I'd known I was going to live this long, I'd have taken better care of myself.

-Jimmy Durante

Facts

1. Diabetes is the sixth leading cause of death in the U.S. among persons ages 75 and older.

2. Estimates suggest that about 20 percent of people ages 65 to 74 in the U.S. have diabetes.

3. It is believed that about one-half of all people with diabetes are unaware of their diagnoses.

4. People with diabetes are two to four times more likely to die from cardiovascular disease than those without diabetes.

5. A Harvard School of Public Health study suggests that men who smoke 25 or more cigarettes each day have roughly double the risk of developing diabetes as nonsmokers.

6. A sedentary lifestyle may contribute to the progression from normal to diabetic ranges of blood sugar levels.

Diabetes mellitus is a leading cause of death and disability among Americans. About seven million people have been diagnosed with diabetes, and an equal number unknowingly have the disease. About 50,000 deaths are attributed to diabetes each year, and the disease contributes to an additional 100,000 deaths each year. Diabetes is the number one cause of end-stage renal disease (ESRD), amputations, and adult blindness in the U.S.

Criteria for the diagnosis of diabetes mellitus have recently been changed. Normal fasting plasma glucose (FPG) is less than 110 mg/dL; the diagnosis diabetes mellitus requires two FPG determinations equal to or greater than 126 mg/dL. Individuals with FPG levels between 110 and 126 are said to have impaired fasting glucose.

Included in the realm of diabetes mellitus and its complications are:

- High levels of sugar in the blood
- Relative or complete insufficiency of insulin, a hormone secreted by the pancreas
- Lack of response or even resistance of certain tissues (liver, muscles) to the action of insulin.
- Premature development of degenerative changes in various tissues and organs
- Complications that lead to various disabling conditions and a shortened life

Patients with Type 1 diabetes mellitus (nine percent of all diabetic patients) have a pancreas with little or no capability of manufacturing insulin. This form of diabetes can occur at any age but most commonly is seen in young children and adolescents.

Patients with Type 2 diabetes mellitus (91 percent of all diabetic patients) retain some capability of producing insulin but show marked resistance or insensitivity to its action. Type 2 patients are often ages 40 or older and are usually overweight and inactive.

Complications seen in both types are similar and are usually related to duration of the disease. Both types can lead to development of:

○ Coronary artery disease
○ Stroke
○ Diseases in the blood vessels of the extremities
○ Nerve disorders
○ Kidney problems
○ Eye problems

Diabetic patients who develop heart attacks or stroke are more likely to develop complications or die from these conditions than are nondiabetic patients. Other complications, such as vision disturbances or complications of treatment (e.g., passing out from low blood sugar), can lead to falls, fractures, and automobile and work-related accidents.

Depression is found in up to 70 percent of patients with diabetic complications and significantly affects the course of the illness. Depressed diabetic patients are less in control of their diets, medications, and exercise programs.

Educating diabetic patients about the disease and the risk factors (i.e., diet, smoking, high blood pressure, high cholesterol, and lack of exercise) that speed its progression or complications can result in extensions of length and quality of life. Recent studies show that in Type 1 diabetic patients, improved blood glucose control can delay significantly the onset and slow the progression of disease-related complications of the kidneys, eyes, and neurological system. Knowledgeable, up-to-date physicians interested in diabetes and skilled in teaching patients can be real assets to patients by overseeing good diabetic control and anticipating and helping prevent complications.

In the U.S., two-thirds of blindness before age 65 is due to diabetes. Because laser therapy has been shown to prevent progression of diabetic retinopathy, diabetic patients should be followed closely by ophthalmologists.

There has been debate for several decades about whether tight blood sugar control alters the course of complications in diabetes. Recently, the question has been answered for Type 1 diabetics who are early in the disease. Specifically, tight blood sugar control with home glucose monitoring and multiple insulin injections per day or insulin pump use has been shown to decrease the onset and progression of eye, kidney, and nerve complications. Studies suggest that elevated blood sugar levels, in a variety of ways, contribute directly to cardiovascular disease. Elevated HbA1c values, used to monitor uncontrolled blood sugars, are associated with a higher incidence of cardiovascular events and deaths. It has been suggested that both types of diabetes would benefit, in terms of microvascular disease and possibly cardiovascular disease, from reductions in HbA1c and that the goal for both types should be a HbA1c of seven percent or less. The particular drug (oral antidiabetic agent or insulin) or drugs used to accomplish this goal appear to be less important than the achievement of the goal itself.

The American Diabetes Association recommends low-dose aspirin (81 to 325 mg per day) to prevent cardiovascular events in diabetics who are ages 30 and older if they have any of the six risk factors for cardiovascular disease or have already been diagnosed with previous cardiovascular events.

Hypertension in both diabetes types is common and accelerates vascular disease. Control of blood pressure, therefore, is important for avoidance of complications. Tight blood pressure control, with a goal of 130/85 mm Hg levels or lower, appears desirable.

Angiotensin-converting enzyme (ACE) inhibitors have been shown to slow progression of eye and kidney disease in Type 1 patients. Because diabetic patients already have vascular disease, smoking increases risks for cardiovascular complications; thus, smoking cessation is important for this population.

Organic erectile dysfunction is common in men with diabetes. Sildenafil (Viagra®) is an effective and well tolerated treatment for this problem. Diabetic patients with coronary artery disease may be at higher risks for complications from this treatment, particularly if they are taking nitrates for angina.

Recommendations
1. Become as knowledgeable as possible about your diabetes.
2. Enlist a physician who is interested in and knowledgeable about diabetes and its complications. You may wish to add an ophthalmologist and a dietician to the team that will oversee your care.

3. Be in control of risk factors that could worsen control or increase complications of your diabetes; risk factors are cigarette smoking, high blood pressure, high cholesterol, obesity, and physical inactivity.
4. Keep your blood pressure level below 130/85 mm Hg.
5. A good exercise program is extremely important.
6. If you have close relatives with diabetes, follow closely the large intervention trials that are aimed at preventing onset of the disease.
7. Watch for the development of symptoms and signs that point to depression and share this information with your physician.

Further Reading

Verge CF and Eisenbarth GS: Strategies for preventing Type I diabetes mellitus. Western J Med;March 1996.

Bone Disease:
How to Avoid Brittle Bones and Fractures

An archeologist is the best husband a woman can have; the older she gets, the more interested he is in her.

-Agatha Christie

Facts

1.   Half of all women in the U.S. and one in eight men will have an osteoporosis-related fracture at some point in their lives.

2.   By age 65, most women lose about 35 percent of their bone mass.

3.   About 15 percent of all women eventually suffer hip fractures.

4.   As many as 20 percent of patients die within a year of hip fracture.

5.   Postmenopausal women who take estrogen supplements for five years can reduce their risks of fractures by about 50 percent.

6.   Women whose mothers had hip fractures before age 80 are about twice as likely to have hip fractures themselves.

7.   Osteoporosis is thought to occur in at least half of patients who receive long-term steroid treatments.

8.   Only a small percentage of patients who take long-term oral cortisone preparations ever receive treatment to prevent or treat osteoporosis.

Few people consider that bone-related problems are factors affecting longevity. Osteoporosis, a bone-thinning disease that leads to increased bone fragility and increased risk of fractures of the hip, spine, wrist, and ribs is found in more than 25 million Americans, 80 percent of whom are women. As many as one of every two women and one in eight men who live past age 80 will have osteoporosis-related fractures. More than one million osteoporosis-related fractures are recorded each year in the U.S. About 70 percent of fractures in individuals ages 45 and older are of the types related to osteoporosis.

Osteoporosis is often thought of as a "silent" disease because bone loss occurs without symptoms and patients have no way of knowing their bones are becoming weak and fragile. The first awareness of osteoporosis may follow a fracture or collapsed vertebra occurring at the time of a fall, sudden strain, or bump.

X-rays can reveal fractures and spinal deformities, but they are not effective for detecting early stages of decreased bone mineral density. Osteoporosis can be diagnosed by bone mineral density testing, which is also valuable for predicting risks of developing fractures and suggesting the need to begin therapy; dual-energy x-ray absorptiometry (DEXA) is a valuable procedure commonly used for these purposes. Bone mineral density testing has been recommended for all women ages 65 and older and those younger than age 65 who have one or more additional risk factors (e.g., menopause, family history, fractures, cigarette smoking, and certain disease processes that cause bone thinning). Because changes in bone mineral density occur slowly with treatment, test results, except in special cases, can best be determined at two-year intervals.

Osteoporotic fracture rates increase significantly with age in both men and women; but at any age, the risk is twice as great in women as men. Elderly white women have about twice the incidence of fractures as African-American women.

Women can lose up to 20 percent of their bone mass in the five to seven years following menopause. This rapid bone loss makes them more susceptible to osteoporosis. Additionally, women have a greater propensity to falling and are more likely than men to survive to the age of vulnerability for falls and fractures.

Osteoporosis is responsible for more than 300,000 hip fractures each year in the U.S., about 840 fractures for every 100,000 persons older than age 65. Hip fractures are not only associated with pain, discomfort, disability, and loss of independence but also have major effects on morbidity and mortality. Estimated expected survival is reduced 15 to 20 percent in the first year after a hip fracture. Though women have more hip fractures than men, the death rate for men within one year of hip fracture is 26 percent higher than that for women. Adding to the problem is the fact that, of individuals living independently prior to a hip fracture, up to 25 percent remain in long-term care institutions a year later.

Causes of osteoporosis are not fully known, though it is known that certain people are more likely to develop the disease than others. Certain modifiable and unmodifiable risk factors are:

Modifiable	**Unmodifiable**
Low-calcium diet	Female sex
Anorexia nervosa or bulimia (forced vomiting)	Advanced age
Smoking	Caucasian or Asian race
Excessive alcohol intake	Small, thin frame
Inactive lifestyle	Family history
Immobilization	Early menopause
Malabsorption of calcium	Abnormal absence of menstrual periods
Low testosterone levels in men	
Endocrine disorders involving thyroid, adrenal, or pituitary glands	
Kidney and liver diseases and certain tumors	
Certain medications	

An important and frequently overlooked risk factor for osteoporosis is use of medications that can lead to bone damage; these include:

- Glucocorticoids (steroids)
- Excessive doses of thyroid hormone
- Seizure medications (e.g., phenytoin [Dilantin®] and barbiturates)
- Aluminum-containing antacids
- Heparin (long-term, high-dose use)
- Certain treatments for endometriosis
- Specialized medicines (e.g., methotrexate, cyclosporin A, cholestyramine)

Long-term oral cortisone preparations commonly used for arthritis, asthma, and chronic lung disease can often result in the development of osteoporosis and spinal and hip fractures. Only a small percentage of patients receiving steroids are on programs to prevent complications. Thus, potential problems should be anticipated or detected early by bone mineral density testing, DEXA being the method of choice. For patients taking steroid medications, the American College of Rheumatology recommends daily intake of 1,500 mg of calcium and at least 800 IU of vitamin D and 30 to 60 minutes per day of weight-bearing exercises. Most patients will need additional treatment in the form of calcitonin, alendronate (Fosamax®), etidronate (Didronel®), estrogen replacement therapy (women), or testosterone therapy (men).

Prevention of osteoporosis is of utmost importance. Adequate diet with sufficient calcium and vitamin D, avoiding smoking, exercising (begun early and continued throughout life), hormone replacement therapy when appropriate or raloxifene (Evista®) in certain settings, and bisphosphonates (e.g., alendronate [Fosamax®]) in people found to be at increased risk all are of proven value. At special risk are Caucasian women older than age 65. A recent study suggests for this population that continuous therapy with low-dose conjugated equine estrogen (0.3 mg per day [Premarin®]) and medroxyprogesterone acetate (2.5 mg per day) along with calcium and vitamin D is a good, effective therapeutic option for prevention of osteoporosis. This combination was well tolerated in this group of women.

Once the diagnosis of osteoporosis is made, the same general measures apply. Calcium and vitamin D supplements may be indicated to ensure adequate intake, and hormone replacement therapy with estrogen and often progesterone added is of proven value. Alendronate (Fosamax®) is useful in treating osteoporosis, as is the naturally occurring hormone, calcitonin (Calcimar®, Miacalcin®), which can be given by injection or nasal spray. Calcitonin is designed to slow bone loss. In recent studies, raloxifene (Evista®) appeared effective in treating and preventing osteoporosis; and a new bisphosphonate, risedronate (Actonel"), appears effective, with claims of fewer gastrointestinal side effects, though it has not yet been FDA-approved for general use.

Approximately one-third of individuals ages 65 and older fall each year. Falls can be due to:

- Various medications that cause:
  - Sedation
  - Lightheadedness
  - Dizziness
  - Loss of balance
  - Lowered blood pressure
- Combinations of medications that present special problems
- Loss of vision
- Loss of hearing
- Muscle weakness
- Loss of coordination
- Diseases that affect balance

Recommendations

1. Be aware of risk factors you may have for osteoporosis.
2. Ensure adequate calcium and vitamin D intake (see chart below).
3. Exercise.
4. Stop smoking.
5. Check with your doctor about medications you take that can cause osteoporosis, especially if you are in a high-risk category.
6. Understand the complications of falls, and institute measures to avoid falling.

7. Make your home a safe environment with adequate lighting, hand rails, and attention to household hazards (e.g., loose carpeting, extension cords, toys).
8. Consider postmenopausal low-dose estrogen therapy.
9. Consider the many new drugs available to prevent and treat osteoporosis.

OPTIMAL CALCIUM AND VITAMIN D REQUIREMENTS

Age Group	Recommended Daily Calcium Intake (mg)
19 to 50	1,000
51 or older	1,200

The average American diet contains only one-third to one-half the recommended daily calcium requirement. It is important that we get as much calcium from our diets as possible (e.g., 8 oz. of skim milk or calcium-fortified orange juice contains 300 mg of calcium). Calcium supplements are available in several forms; they contain varying amounts of elemental calcium, which is the amount of calcium actually available to the body.

Calcium Supplement	Sample Source	Percent of Elemental Calcium	Elemental Calcium in 500 mg Tablet
Calcium carbonate	TUMS	40	200 mg
Calcium citrate	Fortified orange juice	24	120 mg
Calcium gluconate		9	45 mg

Calcium supplements are best taken with meals in single doses of 600 mg or less, which improves absorption. When taken with food, calcium carbonate and calcium citrate are equally well absorbed by the body.

Too much calcium, i.e., 2,500 mg or more per day, can cause problems and prevent the body from getting enough iron, magnesium, and zinc.

Vitamin D is necessary for the body to absorb adequate amounts of calcium. Individuals with low blood levels of vitamin D are at increased risk for fractures due to the development of osteoporosis. Usually, vitamin D needs are met through exposure to sunlight; a daily 10-minute exposure of the hands and face can generate 200 IU of vitamin D. Older people may receive insufficient exposure to sunlight and, in fact, actually require longer exposure times because aging skin is less efficient at producing vitamin D in association with sunlight. Also, elderly populations tend to drink less milk, which is often fortified with vitamin D. Living in northern climates that lack sunlight also adds to this problem, as does use of sunscreens that can block ultraviolet rays needed for vitamin D production.

The recommended daily vitamin D intake is 400 IU for those ages 51 to 70 and 600 IU for those older than age 70. Up to 800 IU and even more has been recommended for the elderly or those at high risk for osteoporosis. Multivitamin preparations often contain about 400 IU.

Dementia:
Not Inevitable in the Elderly

Happiness? That's nothing more than health and a poor memory.

-Albert Schweitzer

Facts

1. At least one-third of individuals who reach age 85 have major impairments of memory and thinking, Alzheimer's disease most often being the cause.

2. Dementia affects up to 15 percent of people ages 65 and older.

3. Dementia may be reversible in approximately 10 percent of patients.

4. Delirium and depression may be misdiagnosed as dementia.

5. Dementia occurs in up to 20 percent of patients with HIV infection.

6. Advanced age and family history are the two most important risk factors for Alzheimer's disease.

7. A large variety and number of drugs lead to memory and/ or thinking impairment.

8. In geriatric clinics, up to 10 percent of those seen for memory problems are found to have reversible dementia related to medications.

Dementia is an acquired loss of memory and/or other mental skills that interfere with the performance of daily activities. Multiple areas of intellectual function are often affected, with areas of impairment including:

- Abstract thinking
- Language
- Judgment
- Perception
- Planning
- Problem-solving
- Memory

Important causes of dementia in older Americans include:

- Alzheimer's disease - 50 to 85 percent
- Vascular disease - 10 to 20 percent, which includes cerebrovascular phenomena such as:
  - Inflammation of blood vessels
  - Emboli or hemorrhages
  - Single or multiple brain infarctions
- Parkinson's disease
- Brain tumors or trauma
- Infections, including:
  - HIV
  - Tuberculosis
  - Syphilis
  - Meningitis
  - Creutzfeldt-Jakob disease
- Metabolic disorders, including:
  - Vitamin B_{12} deficiency
  - Hypothyroidism
- Alcohol abuse
- Poor nutrition

- Medications, either alone or in combination, such as those used for:
  - Pain
  - High blood pressure
  - Sleep
  - Sedation
  - Treatment of psychiatric illnesses

Dementia is responsible for about 120,000 deaths annually, the mortality being strongly associated with its severity. Dementia patients are at increased risk for falls and automobile accidents; as many as 33 percent of demented persons who were still driving had motor vehicle crashes or moving violations within the previous six months of diagnosis, a fact suggesting potential for harm to patients, family members, and care givers as well as to the public.

Dementia is commonly overlooked in its early stages, the time when reversible factors that cause or contribute to the disorder can be managed best. Finding and correcting underlying causes could result in improvement in some patients; such causes include:

- Depression
- Vitamin B_{12} deficiency
- Drug excess or toxicity
- Hypothyroidism
- Alcohol abuse
- Poor nutrition
- Space-occupying lesions (e.g., subdural hematomas)
- Normal pressure hydrocephalus

Common medications often associated with memory impairment or dementia-like situations include steroids, ulcer or heartburn treatment agents, anxiety treatment agents, and sleep medications.

The number of demented patients who experience long-term improvement is relatively small. Some estimates suggest that 10 to 15 percent of dementia patients have a potentially reversible condition (e.g., drug intoxication, depression, or treatable glandular or nutritional disorder). Other studies have shown that about one-half of elderly dementia patients have at least one coexisting illness, the treatment of which could result in improvements for many patients.

It is important that Alzheimer's disease be recognized early because drug therapy can be most effective at this time. Donepezil (Aricept®) appears to improve cognitive function or at least halt cognitive deterioration in many patients with mild or moderate Alzheimer's disease.

Many drugs are being tested for their effectiveness in preventing Alzheimer's disease; these include:

- Nonsteroidal anti-inflammatory drugs (NSAIDs)
- Estrogen
- Vitamin E
- Selegiline
- Steroids
- Colchicine

At this time, these agents are considered to be experimental and, thus, require further careful study before they can be generally recommended.

More commonly used medications can be valuable in treating certain symptoms or associated disorders that are commonly seen with Alzheimer's disease, such as depression, psychosis, and agitation.

Recommendations

1. If you have difficulty with memory, making judgements, or communicating with others, consult your physician or one specializing in dementia.
2. Be familiar with areas of impairment that suggest dementia.
3. When consulting a physician regarding dementia, bring a family member or close friend who is familiar with your day-to-day activities.
4. Check your family history for possible cases of dementia, realizing that diagnosis may have been missed or the symptoms attributed to aging.
5. Don't overlook the possibility of AIDS as a cause of dementia in an elderly patient.

Further Reading

Fleming KC, Adams AC, Petersen RC: Dementia: Diagnosis and evaluation. Mayo Clinic Proceedings, November 1995.

Goldmacher DS and Whitehouse PJ: Evaluation of dementia. N Eng J Med August 1, 1996.

Infections/
HIV and the AIDS Epidemic

The biggest disease today is not leprosy or tuberculosis but rather the feeling of being unwanted.

-Mother Theresa

Facts

1. AIDS is the leading cause of death in the U.S. for those ages 25 to 44.

2. About 10 percent of AIDS cases in the U.S. occur in those ages 50 and older.

3. Estimates suggest that there are approximately one million asymptomatic carriers of the hepatitis B virus in the U.S.

4. Sixty to 80 percent of individuals who use illicit drugs intravenously have evidence of hepatitis B virus infection.

5. Severe pneumococcal bacterial infections result in death in 30 to 40 percent of elderly persons.

6. Influenza is the major cause of death due to infectious disease in the U.S., the last count suggesting 56,000 deaths per year.

At the turn of the twentieth century, the main causes of death in the U.S. were infectious diseases such as influenza, bacterial pneumonia, tuberculosis, and gastrointestinal infections. The development of vaccines and antibiotics, improved hygiene, regulations for food handling, and treated water supplies has led to major inroads in preventing and controlling these diseases; however, new and often difficult to treat infectious agents have proven to be major threats to public health. Viruses, especially HIV, hantavirus, and hepatitis viruses, recently have been of particular concern.

Today, when considering infections that shorten life in significant numbers of people, HIV infection quickly comes to mind. AIDS (acquired immunodeficiency syndrome), a term denoting the later stages of HIV infection with complications, has become the leading cause of death for people ages 25 to 44; recent data suggest that HIV/AIDS is the eighth leading cause of death in the U.S.

AIDS is not only a problem for young adults. About 10 percent of all cases diagnosed each year occur in both genders, ages 50 and older. In certain areas of the country with high concentrations of people older than age 50, this group makes up 14 percent of AIDS cases. Increasing numbers from this group are from heterosexual transmissions and probably are also related to this population's lack of knowledge about HIV infection and its characteristics, diagnosis, and transmission. Unfortunately, the AIDS virus, which can have symptoms such as dementia and weight loss (not uncommon in the elderly), might not even be considered in diagnosing elderly populations.

Current estimates suggest that 650,000 to 900,000 persons in the U.S. are infected with HIV, with approximately 40,000 new infections occurring each year. The vast majority of people infected with HIV will develop AIDS.

According to the Centers for Disease Control and Prevention, men who have sex with men and injection drug users account for more than 80 percent of AIDS cases. Most other cases result from:

- Transmission from mother to fetus
- Sexual partners of injection drug users
- Transfusion of infected blood or blood components

In theory, the virus can be spread by contact with an infected individual's feces, saliva, or urine, though such cases are rare. Individuals at high risk for HIV infection include:

- Men who have sex with men
- Injection drug users
- Sex partners of injection drug users
- Prostitutes and their sex partners
- Homosexual, bisexual, or heterosexual individuals who have had HIV-infected sex partners
- Those who had blood product transfusions between 1978 and 1985
- Those having multiple sex partners, especially if engaging in unprotected sex (i.e., not using latex condoms)

Other infections from bacteria, viruses, and fungi are common throughout life and are found to varying degrees in different age groups. A modest number of infections in the U.S. are associated with a relatively high morbidity and mortality.

Pneumococcal bacterial disease can cause significant morbidity and mortality, especially in the elderly who, through aging, are thought to lose some immunologic functions, making them less able to contain infections. Pneumonia may be difficult to diagnose in the elderly and some cases will be unresponsive or difficult to treat. In some cases, especially hospitalized patients, pneumonia can be prevented by careful feeding and attention to swallowing mechanisms of sick patients and, if possible, by avoiding tubes that assist with feeding or breathing in such patients.

A pneumococcal vaccine appears to be of value, with few adverse effects, for the elderly and especially institutionalized elderly, with the vaccine's protective effect appearing to last five to 10 years.

Influenza can cause significant morbidity and mortality during epidemics. The elderly are at increased risk for the major lethal complications of influenza (i.e., pneumonia). An effective influenza vaccine is available and can reduce mortality associated with influenza outbreaks. For the elderly or other individuals at high risk during a community outbreak, the drugs amantadine (Symmetrel®) and rimantadine (Flumadine®) can be used by those who have not already received the vaccine. A recent FDA-approved drug, zanamivir (Relenza™), which must be inhaled, and not yet approved, oseltamivir (Tamiflu™), which can be given orally when given within 30 hours after the onset of influenza A or B, can reduce the duration of flu-related symptoms and possibly lower the incidence of flu-related complications.

Tuberculosis (TB) rates are increasing in the U.S., especially among African-Americans, Hispanics, and Asians/Pacific Islanders. Up to 15 million persons in the U.S. are infected with the bacteria that causes TB, and foreign-born immigrants are a steady source of new cases. Individuals infected with HIV are more likely to develop active TB than others.

Major problems and increased mortality have been associated with the development of resistance to many of the standard drugs used to treat TB.

Skin tests and chest x-rays can help detect TB infection in exposed individuals who do not have symptoms. Such individuals include:
- Persons infected with HIV
- Persons in close contact with TB patients
- Healthcare workers
- Immigrants
- Residents of long-term care facilities
- Alcoholics
- Illicit drug users

The finding of a newly positive TB skin test reaction is important because a drug, isoniazid, has proven effective in preventing the subsequent development of active TB in such individuals.

Viruses are also the cause of hepatitis B and C, both of which can cause severe liver damage in the form of cirrhosis and liver cancer. As many as 300,000 persons, mostly young adults, become infected with hepatitis B each year, the greatest risk coming from injecting illicit drugs but also commonly from sexual activity.

Healthcare workers are also at risk. A vaccine is available for hepatitis B but not C and should be given to those at increased risks, including:
- Healthcare workers
- Individuals with hemophilia

- Individuals living with infected persons
- Individuals at high risk
- Individuals traveling to parts of the world with a high prevalence of hepatitis B, particularly if engaged in risky behaviors (e.g., sexual activity)

Recommendations

1. Learn basic information about HIV infection and AIDS. Educational material is often provided by hospitals and public health departments.
2. If you are in a high-risk category for HIV infection (i.e., engaged in unprotected sex with a person of unknown HIV status), discuss this situation with your physician and obtain HIV testing.
3. Individuals with new or multiple sex partners should use latex condoms.
4. Seek monogamous sexual relationships with uninfected partners.
5. Patients ages 65 or older, ages 50 or older and living in institutional settings, or having problems such as diabetes, chronic heart or lung disease (emphysema), or chronic kidney problems should obtain pneumococcal vaccines. Patients who have had surgical removal of the spleen or have nonfunctional spleens (sickle cell disease) should obtain pneumococcal vaccines.

Further Reading

Guide to Clinical Preventive Services, Report of the U.S. Preventive Services Task Force, 2nd ed. Williams & Wilkins, 1996.

Sex:
Always a Hot Topic

Really, sex and laughter do go very well together, and I wondered —and still do —which is the more important.

-Hermione Gingold

Facts

1. A high percentage of people experience sexual problems at some time in their lives, but many enjoy sex into their 80s.

2. Numerous medications and recreational drugs can interfere with sexual functioning.

3. Between 20 and 30 million men in the U.S. are consistently unable to have an erection adequate for sexual intercourse.

4. About 85 percent of impotence is due to physical causes, e.g., vascular disease, high blood pressure, diabetes, neurological problems, medications, smoking, or excessive alcohol. About 15 percent is caused by psychological problems.

To date, the authors have found no good studies to indicate that good sex extends life. However, few would deny that good sex throughout life makes life more enjoyable. Good or bad sex is somewhat difficult to define. Probably easiest is to say that the sexual experience depends on whatever the involved couple mutually finds satisfying or unsatisfying.

For satisfying sexual function to occur, there must be a complex interaction of psychological, nervous, vascular, and endocrine systems. Problems involving one of more of those systems interfere with normal sexual function, and the resulting sexual dysfunction can lead to interpersonal problems for the couple, which can worsen the sexual difficulties. The causes of sexual dysfunction are similar in men and women, though the manifestations of sexual dysfunction are more easily recognized in men. Fortunately, most cases of sexual dysfunction are treatable by approaching the underlying physical or psychological problems. It is important, however, that individuals recognize that such problems exist.

The most common problem regarding sexual function in the male is decreased erectile function. For the female, loss of desire for sexual activity is the most common problem and often the most difficult to treat.

Sexual dysfunction, i.e., changes in sexual desire and ability, can be the manifestation of:

- An underlying emotional or psychiatric disorder
- Anxiety
- Stress
- Depression
- Schizophrenia
- Dementia

Professional help from physicians or designated specialists may be needed in many cases. In all cases, thorough histories, physical examinations, and appropriate laboratory evaluations are essential.

Sexual dysfunction may be an early manifestation of an illness that, in one way or another, interferes with interactions of the nervous, vascular, and endocrine systems. Impotence, the inability to achieve an erection adequate for sexual intercourse, is a distressing problem for men that can be caused by a variety of illnesses; recognized disorders include:

- Conditions involving the brain and spinal cord, including:
  - Parkinson's disease
  - Multiple sclerosis
  - Strokes
  - Herniated discs
- Certain blood vessel disorders
- Hypertension
- Coronary artery disease
- Endocrine disorders, including:
  - Diabetes mellitus
  - Thyroid disorders

Low levels of the male hormone testosterone are responsible for only a small percentage of impotence cases. Likewise, menopausal problems or menstrual irregularities are rarely the cause of sexual difficulties in women.

Unfortunately, correction or control of illnesses may not always eliminate sexual dysfunction. However, if the dysfunction is caused by a medication, the problem can often be resolved.

Drugs that interfere with sexual function include:

- High blood pressure medications, including:
  - Diuretics (thiazides, spironolactone)
  - Alphamethyldopa
  - Beta-blockers
  - Hydralazine
  - Reserpine
  - Guanethidine
  - Prazosin
  - Estrogen
- Recreational, abused, or illicit drugs, including:
  - Alcohol
  - Tobacco
  - Cocaine
  - Heroin
  - Opiates
- Antidepressant medications, including:
  - Tricylics (e.g., Elavil®)
  - Monoamine oxidase inhibitors
  - Trazodone
  - Serotonin re-uptake inhibitors (e.g., Prozac®)
- Drugs that act on the central nervous system, including:
  - Phenytoin (Dilantin®)
  - Barbiturates
  - Phenothiazines
- Others, including:
  - Antihistamines/decongestants
  - Cimetidine
  - Cancer chemotherapeutic agents
  - Clofibrate
  - Tranquilizers
  - Digoxin
  - Estrogen

A relatively common recent problem is the use and sometimes abuse of high doses of anabolic steroids by recreational body builders. Use of these agents can be associated with a wide range of serious complications.

The good news for men with impotence (erectile dysfunction) is that most can be helped. Aphrodisiacs do not work; nor do such popular items as ginseng, rhinoceros horn, melatonin, or various other herbs.

In recent years, many new physical methods have been developed for the treatment of erectile dysfunction. A new drug for this problem, sildenafil (Viagra®) has ushered in a new era in the management of erectile dysfunction. Viagra® potentiates the physiological response, causing penile erection after sexual arousal. It appears to be most effective in men who are able to have partial erections and those whose problems have emotional causes, such as depression or anxiety. It can also be effective in men whose problems are due to diabetes or prostate cancer surgery. Though generally a safe drug, Viagra® can be a problem for people with active coronary artery disease, especially those on nitrate medications, those with heart failure and low blood pressures, those on drugs to control blood pressure levels, or those taking certain specific drugs (e.g., erythromycin or cimetidine). Many of the problems associated with this drug occur during or shortly after sexual activity.

Another drug, oral phentolamine (Vasomax®), presently under study, appears to be effective for mild erectile dysfunction and may be of value for patients with cardiovascular problems.

Of interest is the fact that, because erectile

dysfunction is commonly associated with cardiovascular disease, control of cardiovascular risk factors should improve sexual performance; especially important are:

- Exercise
- Diet
- Alcohol restriction
- Not smoking

A study at the University of South Carolina School of Medicine found that men whose total cholesterol levels were greater than 240 mg/dL were almost twice as likely to become impotent as those whose cholesterol levels were below 180 mg/dL. Studies at Duke University also suggest that cholesterol-blocked vessels may slow the flow of blood to the penis, which contributes to impotence.

Unfortunately, research on female sexual dysfunction has not been as productive as that for males. At present, there are no effective drugs for the treatment of sexual dysfunction in females, although sildenafil (Viagra®) is under investigation. Early and relatively small studies of Viagra® in postmenopausal women do not suggest improved sexual function with its use. Some drugs, such as androgens, are also being evaluated for female sexual dysfunction problems. Many women seek hormone replacement therapy to reverse sexual difficulties; in some cases, such therapy can be effective. There is some evidence, however, that the addition of progesterone can blunt the positive effects of estrogen therapy.

A common source of anxiety related to sexual activity occurs after a heart attack or coronary bypass surgery. The concern is that sexual intercourse may trigger another heart attack. However, studies suggest that heart attack patients who are otherwise doing well have little, if any, risk from sexual intercourse and should be able to resume sexual activity during the second week after hospital discharge. One recognized source of increased risk, however, is having sex with a person other than the usual partner.

It has been suggested that sexual intercourse as an exercise might be the equivalent of climbing about 20 stairs. If this is true, it is better understood why sexual activity as an exercise factor, or cholesterol burner, does not contribute to life extension. On the other hand, a happy wife is more likely to see that her husband gets his five servings of fruits and vegetables daily, avoids depression, takes his medications, and visits his doctor.

Recommendations

1. If you experience sexual dysfunction problems, do not hesitate to seek professional help.
2. Communicate to your partner the sexual feelings and behaviors in which you would like to engage.
3. Remember that certain diseases and various drugs can cause sexual dysfunction.
4. Most couples eventually experience some form of sexual problems that can be satisfactorily resolved by knowledgeable, caring physicians.
5. Ask your physician about trying Viagra® for your erectile dysfunction.

Injuries/Accidents/ Domestic Violence

With a good heredity, nature deals you a fine hand at cards; and with good environment, you learn to play the hand well.
                                    -Walter C. Alvarez, M.D.

Facts

1. Injury is the third leading cause of death in the U.S.

2. Motor vehicle crash-related injuries are the eighth leading cause of death in the U.S.

3. Falls are the second leading cause of unintentional injury death in the U.S.

4. Smoking materials have been implicated in up to 33 percent of residential fire deaths among the elderly.

5. Increased use of automobile safety restraints contributed to a 32-percent decline in the death rate from car crashes.

6. Domestic violence is the leading cause of injury to women in the U.S., with an estimated 4,000 women killed each year. Battering accounts for about one-half of all serious injuries in women presenting to emergency departments.

7. When compared with nonsmokers, smokers are 1.5 times more likely to have motor vehicle crashes, 1.4 to 2.5 times more likely to be injured at work, and twice as likely to suffer other unintentional injuries.

Injury is an important cause of death in the U.S., accounting each year for about 4.3 million potential years of life lost prematurely before age 70. Injuries are not necessarily accidents, i.e., those that occur by chance and are unavoidable, because they usually can be attributed to preventable behavioral and environmental factors. Important causes of injuries include:

- Motor vehicle crashes
- Burns
- Drowning
- Poisoning
- Falls

Injuries commonly occur in the workplace. In the U.S., 17 work-related fatalities occur each day; their leading causes* are:

- Motor vehicles - 23 percent
- Machines - 13 percent
- Homicides - 12 percent
- Falls - 10 percent
- Electrocutions - 7 percent
- Strikes by falling objects - 7 percent
- All others - 28 percent

*(From *For a Healthy Nation*, U.S. Department of Health and Human Services, Public Health Service)

Motor vehicle crash-related injuries are important causes of death. Motor vehicle fatality rates are highest for the young and elderly. Drivers ages 70 and older have more fatalities than middle-aged drivers; these fatalities are related to:

- Loss of vision
- Loss of hearing
- Dulled reaction times

Dementia particularly impairs driving ability, as do alcohol and sleep disorders.

All drivers should recognize the values of:

- Seat belts
- Helmets (bicycle or motorcycle)
- Air bags
- Periodic vision and hearing exams
- Driving free of the influence of:
  - Alcohol
  - Illicit drugs
  - Certain over-the-counter medications
  - Certain prescription medications

Many medications have mind-altering effects. About one-third of drivers killed in crashes are intoxicated by alcohol. Drunk drivers are at a disadvantage because their driving skills are impaired, they are less likely to use seat belts, and they are more likely to speed. Drugs such as marijuana, cocaine, and tranquilizers are also important contributors to lethal crashes.

Wearing a seat belt can increase the survival rate of car crash passengers by one-half. Those thrown from vehicles are 24 to 40 times more likely to be killed. Frontal air bags can potentially reduce risks of death by an additional nine percent among belted drivers and 20 percent among unbelted front-seat passengers. Your physician may comment and advise you on habits, physical or mental deficiencies, or prescribed medications that can hamper your ability to drive or operate machines that require significant skill and attention.

At least one-third of older adults fall each year in the U.S., resulting in about 12,000 deaths. Falls by elderly people lead to injuries, such as hip fractures, which, in turn, result in death 10 to 20 percent of the time. Among the elderly, hip fractures are the most frequent serious consequence of falling; approximately 20 percent of falls result in direct impact on the hip. Wearing protective pads can significantly reduce risks of hip fractures in this group.

Some environmental risk factors can be corrected to help prevent falls; these include:
- Pavement irregularities
- Slippery floors
- Poor lighting
- Poorly-fitting shoes or inadequate shoe size

Helping to protect against falls, especially for the elderly, are:
- Weight-bearing exercise training
- Gait retraining
- Gait aids
- Adequate vision correction
- Recognition of medication side effects

Combinations of these efforts can reduce risks of falling by about 30 percent.

Burn injuries, most commonly flame and scald injuries, have the highest mortality for those ages 60 and older. Cigarette smoking is an important cause of fire and burn injury deaths and is associated with about 25 percent of residential fires. Homes often do not have smoke detectors; additionally, elderly patients may not be able to hear or respond to alarms. Avoiding smoking, especially in bed, and attention to the temperatures of tap water, food, and drinks can greatly reduce the incidence of fire and burn injuries.

Unintentional poisonings lead to a significant number of deaths among adults, the highest incidence being in young adult men. Most of these deaths are related to overdose of alcohol or drugs such as heroin and cocaine. Elderly patients with arthritis or other painful problems may excessively use aspirin and/or other pain relievers that can lead to:

- Gastrointestinal bleeding
- Confusion
- Kidney failure
- Pulmonary edema

In the U.S. each year, four to eight million women from all cultural and socioeconomic groups suffer physical abuse inflicted by their spouses or partners. Adult women are more likely to be sexually assaulted, beaten, and killed in their own homes at the hands of their male partners than any place else or by anyone else in society.

Estimates also suggest that up to two million cases of elder abuse occur annually in the U.S. This is of particular concern as the population ages. The mistreatment of the elderly may be even more difficult to identify because of:

- The relative isolation of this group
- The tendency not to report this form of abuse
- The subtle forms that this abuse can take so that it is often undetected

Help for such victims involves community efforts that include individuals, agencies, healthcare facilities, and law enforcement organizations that are motivated to work together for the reduction and prevention of violence. Victims should understand that they can initiate help simply by calling 911. Getting to a hospital emergency room will also initiate desired assistance.

Recommendations

1. If you have been drinking alcoholic or using mind-altering drugs, do not drive or operate potentially dangerous machinery.
2. If you have difficulty walking or have frequent falls, inform your physician, who will look for and work to correct reversible causes.
3. Do not smoke, especially in bed.
4. Be sure to have periodic vision and hearing tests.
5. Always wear a seat belt or helmet (motorcycle or bicycle).
6. Recognize that medicines you take may have potential mind-altering effects.
7. Learn what facilities your community has for aiding victims of domestic violence.

Further Reading

Scheitel SM, Fleming KC, Chutha DS, Evans JM: Geriatric Health Maintenance, Mayo Clinic Proceedings, March 1966.

Guide to Clinical Preventive Services, Report of the U.S. Preventive Services Task Force, 2nd ed. Williams & Wilkins, 1996.

The Bad (Polypharmacy) and the Ugly (Cocaine)

There are some remedies worse than the disease.

-Pubblius Syrus

Facts

1. Elderly Americans (ages 65 and older) account for 30 percent of all prescription and 40 percent of all over-the-counter drug purchases.

2. Age-related changes in elderly patients allow drugs to maintain their effects longer, have unusual or unexpected actions, and cause more adverse reactions with serious or potentially life-threatening outcomes.

3. The average nursing home patient receives four to seven different medications daily.

4. Cocaine-related injuries are a major cause of death among young adults in areas such as New York City.

5. A heart attack is the most commonly reported cardiac complication of cocaine abuse.

6. Chest pain is the most common cocaine-related medical problem, resulting in the evaluation of more than 64,000 patients annually for possible coronary artery problems.

During the last 30 years, the number of FDA-approved drugs available for the treatment of diseases and their medical complications has increased from 650 to more than 9,500, and of those there are approximately 1,000 generic compounds. The shear volume of drugs makes it impossible, without the aid of sophisticated computer systems, for physicians to master knowledge of the complex actions of specific drugs, their complications, their interactions with other drugs, and their altered activities in various disease states. Fortunately, recent developments have made more drug information available so that physicians may keep abreast of the latest findings.

Polypharmacy

The seriousness of problems related to adverse drug events is apparent, considering that:

- Prescription-related drug problems result in about 119,000 annual U.S. deaths.
- Twenty-eight percent of hospitalized patients experience adverse drug events, translating to 8.8 million hospitalizations each year.
- Tens of thousands of fatalities in hospitalized patients in the U.S. occur annually due to drugs.
- One in four people ages 65 and older receive at least one of 20 drugs that are potentially inappropriate for elderly patients.
- Thirty percent of elderly patients use eight or more prescription drugs daily, and the elderly population takes an average of 18 prescription drugs per year.

- It is estimated that 10 to 30 percent of hospital admissions among the elderly are related to drug problems such as:
  - Inappropriate drug prescribing
  - Noncompliance
  - Adverse drug events

Elderly people are especially prone to adverse drug events because of their intakes of multiple medications, use of herbal preparations unknown to their physicians, and incidences of multiple chronic diseases. This problem is of particular concern because the elderly population is expected to increase from 31 million in 1989 to 52 million in the year 2020.

Cocaine

In a particular year, more than four million Americans use cocaine, with about one-third of those using the drug monthly. Though figures are difficult to determine, it has been estimated that more than 20 million Americans have tried cocaine at least once.

Cocaine can cause problems no matter what the route of administration (intranasal, smoking, or intravenous injection) and can be directly related to a variety of problems, including:

- Heart attacks
- Seizures
- Respiratory distress
- Mental problems
- Muscle necrosis and renal failure

Indirectly, cocaine can be associated with:

- Homicides
- Suicides
- Motor vehicle accidents

Heart attacks are the most commonly reported cardiac complication of cocaine use. Even small amounts of the drug can trigger an event, even in the first-time user. Heart attacks can occur shortly after use or on the following day and can occur in a young person with normal coronary arteries, suggesting the occurrence of spasm and occlusion of a coronary artery. The risk of heart attack is tremendously increased in the 60 minutes following cocaine use.

Cocaine can also cause sudden death by other mechanisms, such as:

- Heart rhythm disturbances
- Strokes
- Sudden major increases in blood pressure

Besides the drug itself, certain adulterants found in street cocaine can present major problems.

Recommendations

1. At least once a year, bag all your pills, take them to your doctor, and ask if you still need all of them and if there are any you can do without.
2. Remember that a medication (or combination of medications) you take could explain a worsening of your condition, new symptoms, or even a new illness.
3. Learn as much as you can about your medications. Elderly patients should ask for help (from family, friends, caregivers) with this sometimes burdensome task.
4. Be sure to inform your physician of any herbal preparations you are taking.
5. NEVER, EVER, USE ANY FORM OF COCAINE.
6. If already dependent on cocaine, seek the assistance of your physician or a substance-abuse specialist.

Smoking:
Enormous Complications of Addiction and Powerful Benefits from Quitting

Tobacco drieth the brain, dimmeth the sight, vitiateth the smell, hurteth the stomach, destroyeth the concoction, disturbeth the humors and spirits, corrupteth the breath, induceth a trembling of the limbs, exiccateth the windpipe, lungs and liver, annoyeth the milt, scorcheth the heart, and causeth the blood to be adjusted.

- Tobias Venner

Facts

1. An average smoker dies eight years earlier than a nonsmoker.

2. Studies suggest that 30 to 40 percent of the half million yearly U.S. deaths from coronary artery disease are due to smoking.

3. Smoking only one to four cigarettes a day can more than double the risk of death from coronary artery disease.

4. Smoking is the cause of 30 percent of all deaths from cancer.

5. When you smoke, everyone around you smokes.

6. Female nonsmokers who are regularly exposed to others' smoke are 91-percent more likely to have heart attacks than those not exposed.

7. Nonsmokers living with smokers have a 30-percent higher risk of dying from heart disease than nonsmokers without such exposure.

8. Cigarette smoking is the number one preventable cause of premature death in the U.S.

9. A 40-year study of British physicians has predicted that about half of all regular smokers will eventually die as a result of cigarette use.

10. Cigarette smoking is the leading risk factor for age-related macular degeneration, the leading cause of blindness in people older than age 65.

Smoking and other tobacco use methods have been chosen as the first risk factors discussed in this book because they best exemplify the concept that is hoped to be relayed to readers: one's life can be extended significantly by certain reasonable actions. The best and most recent data indicate that smoking-related illnesses account for nearly one in five deaths and more than one-fourth of all deaths among those ages 35 to 64. It has been estimated that during the 1990s in developed countries, tobacco use will cause about 30 percent of all deaths among this age group, making smoking the largest single cause of premature death in the developed world.

In the U.S., according to the best recent estimate, when those who die from passive smoking (the breathing of sidestream smoke emitted from burning tobacco) are included, tobacco kills about 480,000 people each year and causes about 180,000 deaths each year from cardiovascular disease (i.e., coronary artery disease and stroke).

Heart disease, not cancer, is the main disease caused by smoking. Though heavy smoking for long periods is generally recognized as a problem, smokers tend to ignore studies that show that lesser exposures can also be lethal. In one major study of nurses, it was found that those who smoked one to four cigarettes daily had a 2.5-fold increased risk of fatal coronary artery disease and nonfatal heart attack when compared to nurses who did not smoke. Some individuals are so sensitive to tobacco smoke that the mere entrance into a smoke-filled room can cause their coronary arteries to go into spasm, occlude blood flow, and cause chest pain and possible damage to the heart muscle.

Cigarette smoking is responsible for 30 percent of all deaths from cancer and represents the most important preventable cause of cancer in the U.S. Besides causing 85 percent of lung cancer cases, smoking is also associated with cancers of the:

- Mouth
- Throat
- Larynx
- Esophagus
- Stomach
- Pancreas
- Cervix
- Kidney
- Ureter
- Bladder
- Colon

As occurs with heart disease, cancer, in certain unfortunate individuals, can be caused by short periods of exposure to relatively small numbers of cigarettes. Passive smoking, such as exposure to parents' smoke during childhood and adolescence as well as exposure from living with a spouse who smokes or working with fellow employees who smoke, is also a recognized cause of lung and other cancers. Cigarette smoking is also the leading cause of lung illness and death in the U.S., causing more than 84,000 deaths annually from such problems as:

- Emphysema
- Pneumonia
- Bronchitis

Problems related to use of tobacco products are present at each and every age of life. An article in *Time* magazine reported that even three insurance firms owned by tobacco companies charge smokers nearly double the premiums for term life insurance because smokers are about twice as likely to die at any given age.

The hazards of smoking extend well into later life. Among those older than age 65, the rates of total mortality among current smokers are twice those of people who never smoked. Oral cancer in men who use smokeless tobacco (e.g., snuff, chewing tobacco) typically occur in the older than age 65 group, though it can be seen much earlier.

The recent resurgence of cigar smoking overlooks the fact that there is no safe form of tobacco, just as there is no safe period of time for tobacco use. Estimates of deaths from pipe and cigar smoking just prior to the recent increase in cigar sales were 14,000 yearly in the U.S. The popularity of cigars among young people is in part related to the belief that cigars are a safe alternative to cigarettes. However, a report from the National Cancer Institute suggests that people who smoke cigars daily have about the same risk for oral, laryngeal, and esophageal cancers as cigarette smokers. Also, cigars give off thick clouds of secondhand smoke containing similar cancer-causing substances as cigarettes, though in considerably higher concentrations.

Even cigar smokers who do not inhale are exposed to their own environmental tobacco smoke, and smoke, of course, is definitely a risk factor for coronary artery disease and emphysema. Previous cigarette smokers who turn to cigars are more likely to inhale than those who have not smoked cigarettes. It would not be unusual for a cigar smoker to take in more nicotine and other smoke toxins than a cigarette smoker, depending on the person's manner of smoking and the type of cigar smoked. Regular cigar smokers have a significantly increased risk of lung cancer as well as coronary artery disease. More study is needed to determine the health risks of the occasional cigar smoker.

Many smokers are switching to lower tar and nicotine cigarette brands rather than quitting, in the misguided belief that they can smoke more safely. A wealth of scientific evidence contradicts this strategy, however, because smokers inhale these low-yield cigarettes more deeply and smoke more of them to obtain the same nicotine kick.

Those fortunate enough to escape death from tobacco toxin exposure can still find themselves compromised in later life by damaged hearts or emphysematous lungs. These and other consequences of tobacco-related injuries can make afflicted individuals more at risk for other illnesses (e.g., pneumonia, stroke) common to later life.

Much still can be gained by those who, after any period of using any quantity or variety of tobacco (cigarettes, cigars, pipes, snuff, or chewing tobacco) at any age, are able to kick the habit, provided the lethal condition has not yet become manifest:

- After about a year, mortality from heart disease drops halfway back to that of nonsmokers and after five years to the rate equal to nonsmokers.
- Risk of lung cancer is cut in half in five years and approaches that of nonsmokers after about 15 years.

- Lifelong smokers who quit at age 50 double their chances of living to age 65.
- Smokers who die between ages 35 and 64 lose 23 years of life compared to age-matched nonsmokers.

Today smokers are quitting in large numbers with the help of sympathetic physicians and through use of or help from:

- Nicotine patches and gums (which can be purchased over-the-counter)
- Nicotine nasal spray (Nicotrol® NS)
- Nicotine inhaler (Nicotrol® Inhaler)
- Bupropion (Zyban®)
- Behavior modification programs
- Effective medicines for associated anxiety
- The almost daily reports in the media regarding the dangers of tobacco
- Acknowledgements of subversive activities of the tobacco industry

The nicotine nasal spray has the advantage of delivering nicotine more rapidly than gum, patches, or inhalers but not nearly as rapidly as cigarettes. The nicotine inhaler has added effectiveness because it simulates the habitual hand-to-mouth action that is so common to smoking. Bupropion (Zyban®), an extended-release antidepressant, appears to work for smokers regardless of histories of depression. It also appears, in some individuals, to lessen the problem of weight gain that is often related to quitting smoking. All these drugs, by themselves or in combination, especially when accompanied by behavioral support, have value in helping people quit smoking and remain tobacco-free.

For those who find cost to be a factor, an inexpensive antidepressant, nortriptyline, may be effective for nondepressed smokers. Also on the horizon is a nicotine lollipop, which addresses the oral gratification aspect of smoking.

A recent study suggests that participation in regular, vigorous physical exercise facilitates smoking cessation in women. The exercise program, in conjunction with a cognitive-behavioral smoking cessation program, not only facilitated smoking cessation but also delayed weight gain in women smokers and improved exercise capacity. Such a program could be a valuable addition to all smoking cessation programs.

Recommendations
1. If you are a smoker, quit. If you chew tobacco, stop.
2. If you live with a smoker, discuss your concerns for your health with him/her and review data together. Your goal should be that smokers not smoke in your presence or in rooms that you frequent or, if possible, anywhere in your house. Tobacco toxins have tremendous capabilities of moving from room to room and from one floor to another.
3. If you are exposed to passive smoke at work, discuss your concerns with fellow employees or your boss. It may be necessary to change jobs. Your personal physician may be able to document your distress or risks from such exposure. Studies have shown added risks for those exposed to passive smoking both at home and at work.
4. For help quitting smoking, seek the assistance of your physician or a physician skilled in

smoking cessation programs. Because smokers have more depression, physicians may detect and treat this in the process of supporting their patients' tobacco cessation programs.

5. Tips for individuals who require extra assistance in quitting are listed below.

Further Reading

Bartecchi CE, MacKenzie TD, Schrier RW: The human cost of tobacco use. New Eng J Med March 31 and April 7, 1994.

Bartecchi CE, MacKenzie TD, Schrier RW: The global tobacco epidemic. Sci Am May 1995.

Clearing the Air: How to Quit Smoking and Quit for Keeps. Prepared by the Office of Cancer Communications, National Cancer Institute. NIH Publication No. 89-1647, February 1989.

Smoking Facts and Tips for Quitting. National Institutes of Health, National Cancer Institute. NIH Publication No. 93-3405, September 1993.

Tips to Help You Stop Smoking

Patients should realize that approximately 40 million Americans have quit smoking and that about 95 percent of these stopped on their own without any formal cessation program. Quitting rates are about twice as high for those who quit on their own as for those who participate in formal smoking cessation programs.

Of the various strategies for quitting, those who do so "cold turkey" are more likely to remain abstinent. Ongoing encouragement and assistance from physicians has also been cited by successful quitters as important in their decisions to quit and in preventing relapses.

Those who want to quit smoking should realize that some short-term discomforts/withdrawal symptoms will occur; these include:

- Dry mouth
- Sore throat
- Sore gums
- Sore tongue
- Headache
- Trouble sleeping
- Fatigue
- Hunger
- Tenseness
- Irritability
- Coughing

These symptoms peak within a few days but usually last only a week or two. Relapses can occur in the first week after quitting and even for months afterwards, and these can be particularly hard times. Slips may occur, especially during periods of emotional turmoil, but should not be equated with total failure. It is important to keep trying. Many successful quitters failed repeatedly before they were finally able to quit.

A great deal of experience with smokers and their efforts to quit has led organizations such as the National Institutes of Health, the National Cancer Institute, and the American Heart Association to recommend the following tips to help smokers in their efforts to quit.

GETTING READY TO QUIT

1. Select a target date for quitting, possibly a special day, such as a birthday, anniversary, or holiday.
2. Decide positively that you want to quit. Try to avoid negative thoughts about how difficult it might be.
3. List all the reasons why you want to quit. Write them down and carry them with you. Read them whenever you are tempted to smoke.
4. Notice when and why you smoke. Try to find the things in your daily life that you often do while smoking, such as drinking your morning cup of coffee or talking on the telephone.
5. Change your smoking routines. Keep your cigarettes in a different place, or make them difficult to find. Smoke with your other hand.
6. Smoke only in certain places, such as outdoors, or in places that are uncomfortable.
7. Begin to condition yourself physically. Start a modest exercise program, drink more fluids, get plenty of rest, and avoid fatigue.
8. Choose your environment. Spend more and more time in places where smoking is not allowed.
9. Ask your spouse or a friend to quit with you. Share your feelings and offer mutual support.
10. Switch to a brand of cigarettes you find distasteful.
11. Collect all your cigarette butts in one large glass container to remind yourself of the filth that smoking represents. Don't empty your ashtrays. This will remind you how many cigarettes you smoke each day.
12. Smoke only those cigarettes you really want. Catch yourself before you light up a cigarette out of pure habit.
13. Think of quitting in terms of one day at a time.

THE DAY YOU QUIT

1. Throw away all your cigarettes and matches. Put away your lighters and ashtrays.

2. Change your morning routine. When you eat breakfast, sit at a different place at the table. Stay busy, exercise, or go to the movies.

3. When you get the urge to smoke, do something else instead. Try to replace the urge by chewing sugarless gum or mints. Snack on celery or carrots.

4. Remind family and friends that this is your quit date and ask for their help over the next couple of weeks.

5. Carry other things to put in your mouth, such as gum, hard candy, or a toothpick.

6. Spend this day and following days with nonsmokers and in places where smoking is not allowed.

7. Drink large quantities of water and fruit juices (avoid caffeine beverages).

8. Avoid alcohol, coffee, or other beverages that you associate with cigarette smoking.

9. If you miss the sensation of having a cigarette in your hand, play with something else, such as a pencil, paper clip, or marble.

10. Visit your dentist and have your teeth cleaned to get rid of tobacco stains.

11. Reward yourself at the end of the day. Estimate the amount of money you saved and buy yourself a treat, such as a movie or a book, and enjoy your favorite meal.

12. Limit your socializing to healthful, outdoor activities and sports in situations in which it would be difficult to smoke.

13. Don't allow yourself to think that "one cigarette won't hurt". It will!

STAYING OFF CIGARETTES

1. Don't worry if you are sleepier or more short-tempered than usual. These feelings will pass.
2. Begin to increase your exercise program.
3. Review in your mind the positive things about quitting, such as how much you like yourself as a nonsmoker and the health benefits to you and your family. A positive attitude can help through rough times.
4. When you feel tense, try to keep busy. Think about ways to solve the problem, tell yourself smoking won't make it any better, and do something else.
5. Eat regular meals. Feeling hungry is sometimes mistaken for the desire to smoke.
6. Start a money jar with the money you save by not buying cigarettes.
7. Let others know you quit smoking. Most people will support you.
8. If you slip and smoke, don't be discouraged. Many former smokers tried to stop several times before they finally succeeded. Quit again.
9. Watch your food and calorie intake so as not to gain weight during this period. Count calories if necessary. Increased exercise can help burn calories.
10. Follow-up visits with your physician, usually at the end of the second week, may prove helpful. Further help in the form of extra motivation, advice, and/or nicotine gum or patches might be suggested or instituted.
11. Watch out for triggers that are commonly recognized as stimulating a sudden, intense urge to smoke, such as:
    ○ Working under pressure
    ○ Feeling blue
    ○ Talking on the telephone
    ○ Having a drink
    ○ Watching television

- Driving your car
- Finishing a meal
- Playing cards
- Drinking coffee
- Watching someone else smoke

12. When possible, support new taxes that raise the price of cigarettes, making the smoking habit even more painful.
13. Periodically, write down new reasons why you're happy you quit and post these where you'll be sure to see them.

This extensive, though not exhaustive list is not meant to be burdensome to the potential quitter. The authors recommend reviewing the list and selecting those items you can implement successfully, realizing that all have value and have proven effective for some individuals.

Good and Bad Cholesterol: Implications for Cardiovascular Disease

As I see it, every day you do one of two things: build health or produce disease in yourself.

-Adelle Davis

Facts

1. At any cholesterol level, a 10-percent increase in serum cholesterol is associated with a 20-percent or greater increased risk of coronary artery disease.

2. A 10-percent reduction in serum cholesterol could result in as much as a 10-percent reduction in death from coronary artery disease.

3. About 40 million Americans are thought to have cholesterol levels high enough to require medical attention.

4. Studies suggest that only 45 to 65 percent of patients with high cholesterol had evidence of treatment.

5. Newer drugs that have been shown to lower cholesterol in patients with cardiovascular disease also have been shown to prolong life significantly.

6. The newer drugs, commonly called statins, not only have the ability to decrease the risk of the first or subsequent heart attack or stroke but also have the capacity to prevent such problems from occurring at all.

7. At present, for cholesterol problems in persons ages 75 and older, there are not enough data to determine the value of screening or treatment.

Cholesterol is a soft, waxy, fat-like substance that is produced only by animals, is normally found throughout the body, and is necessary for healthy body function. The substance becomes a problem when too much is present and is deposited in the wrong places, such as in the coronary arteries or arteries leading to the brain or blood vessels in the legs.

Cholesterol travels throughout the body in the bloodstream packaged in units called lipoproteins:

- Low-density lipoprotein (LDL), also known as bad cholesterol, is the main cholesterol-carrying compound in the blood. It plays an important role in plaque formation within arteries
- High-density lipoprotein (HDL), also known as good cholesterol, helps remove cholesterol from arteries and transports it to the liver for clearance from the bloodstream
- Very low-density lipoprotein (VLDL) transports triglycerides to the tissues where they are broken down and used for energy or are stored. Triglyceride formation is increased when excess calories are present

Some people inherit a disorder that results in high cholesterol levels and early-onset, severe coronary artery disease. Others have cholesterol problems due to lifestyle choices such as poor diet, inactivity, or smoking. Some have combinations of these entities.

Levels of fats in the blood can be determined by direct measurements or formulae. The total cholesterol measurement, the most common test, is made up of LDL, HDL, and other blood lipid particle levels. Some helpful numbers to remember for individuals without known heart disease are:

Cholesterol Types	Levels (mg/dL)		
	Desirable	**Borderline**	**Undesirable**
Total cholesterol	Less than 200	200 to 239	Greater than 240
HDL cholesterol	Greater than 45	35 to 44	Less than 35
LDL cholesterol	Less than 130	130 to 160	Greater than 160
Triglycerides	Less than 200	200 to 400	Greater than 400

Even stricter goals are set for those with known heart disease. A recent study of heart attack patients suggests there is considerable benefit derived from treatment with lipid-lowering drugs, even if LDL cholesterol is not above 130. Such treatment could involve as many as four million people. Many specialists even recommend using a statin drug to treat all coronary artery disease patients with LDL cholesterol levels above 100 unless these patients have contraindications to taking such drugs.

At present, there is much controversy about who should be screened for high cholesterol. Physicians will inform their patients about which tests are needed, when they are needed, and how patients should prepare for them. Certainly those at risk for coronary artery disease, those who have suffered heart attacks, and middle-aged men with cardiac risk factors are in need of screening studies. Family or personal histories of cholesterol or vascular problems (e.g., stroke) also suggest benefit from screening. Abnormal cholesterol studies are of less value in persons ages 70 years and older unless they are known to have coronary artery disease.

Finding elevated total blood cholesterol in young or middle-aged individuals suggests the need to measure other lipoprotein levels. For those at risk, the higher the total cholesterol level, the greater the risk of cardiovascular disease. This risk is further increased if LDL is high and HDL is low, a particularly bad combination. Under any circumstances, however, high LDL is undesirable because it causes atherosclerosis. However, low HDL by itself is also of concern. We must also keep in mind that individuals with high HDL levels can still have heart attacks.

For age groups at risk for coronary artery disease, the lower the LDL and higher the HDL, the less likely it is that heart attacks will occur. Abnormal cholesterol tests, when combined with other risk factors, increase significantly the risks of developing cardiovascular disease. Other risk factors are:

◎ High blood pressure
◎ Diabetes
◎ Age
◎ Male gender
◎ Smoking
◎ Obesity
◎ Family history
◎ Lack of exercise
◎ Lower socioeconomic status

The presence of several risk factors further magnifies the problem in such individuals. Those who are placed in the high-risk group due to the combination of cholesterol tests and risk factors should seek their physicians' help to outline programs for cholesterol control and risk factor reduction. It is suggested that for each one-percent reduction in blood cholesterol, there may be a two-percent reduction in heart attack risk.

Less can be said about triglycerides, mainly because the data are not complete about this fat. It is known that triglycerides can be elevated in diabetes and thyroid, liver, and kidney diseases. Certain drugs, even oral estrogens in some women, and alcohol in excess can also raise triglyceride levels. It is especially important that triglycerides be measured while fasting because a recent meal or even a cup of coffee can raise triglyceride levels.

High plasma triglyceride levels on their own or especially in combination with other cholesterol problems appear to be associated with coronary artery disease, and very high triglyceride levels can precipitate bouts of pancreatitis. In any case, elevated triglycerides should indicate:

○ Weight loss for obese patients
○ Dietary manipulation
○ Exercise
○ Reduction of alcohol intake

Some individuals may require drug treatment. Good programs are available for control of abnormal cholesterol levels; however, diet and exercise should form the basis of any program. Weight loss for obese patients is definitely helpful; increasing fiber intake can lower cholesterol levels. For postmenopausal women, adding estrogen can lower cholesterol levels.

Because low HDL levels are associated with greater risks of coronary artery disease, it is advantageous to attempt to raise HDL levels. This can be accomplished through:

○ Exercise
○ Weight loss
○ Stopping smoking

○ Estrogen replacement therapy
○ Moderate alcohol drinking
○ Dietary changes, especially eating lesser amounts of foods containing trans-fats and replacing dietary calories from carbohydrates with those from unsaturated fats
○ Some drug therapies, e.g., niacin

The value of lowering "bad", or LDL, cholesterol is now unquestioned. Reducing LDL levels not only decreases the number of recurrent events in heart patients but also prevents coronary artery disease in persons at low to moderate risk of developing the problem. Lowering LDL levels has been shown to reduce just about every clinical manifestation of the atherosclerotic process, i.e., reducing:

○ Total mortality
○ Fatal and nonfatal heart attack incidences
○ Incidence of stroke
○ Unstable angina pectoris
○ Peripheral vascular disease (even to the mid-70s)

The program to lower LDL levels should begin with diet and exercise, especially in combination; if overweight is evident, achieving a desirable weight range is indicated. Employing a diet such as the American Heart Association's Step 1 or Step 2 diets under tight supervision (i.e., within hospital metabolic ward) can reduce blood cholesterol (mostly LDL) by up to 15 percent, though less than half that reduction can be expected in free-living subjects. Dietary modifications, such as replacing some saturated fats with monounsaturated fats or omega–3 fatty acids, increasing fruits and vegetables for their antioxidant properties, increasing dietary fiber, and avoiding trans-fatty acids, all have value.

Although use of specific diets can be effective, it is often difficult for people to comply with some programs, especially for the long-term. Certain products, especially those containing plant sterols and stanols derived from foods, are capable of lowering cholesterol by reducing the amount of cholesterol that gets absorbed by the gut; these are being developed and are making their way to the marketplace.

If desired LDL cholesterol levels cannot be achieved by these methods, use of a group of cholesterol lowering drugs, statins, is in order. These agents have been associated with a 50-percent or greater decrease in LDL levels, a tendency to increase "good" HDL levels, and an ability to lower triglyceride levels.

Presently there are six statin drugs:
- Atorvastatin (Lipitor®)
- Cerivastatin (Baycol™)
- Fluvastatin (Lescol®)
- Lovastatin (Mevacor®)
- Pravastatin (Pravachol®)
- Simvastatin (Zocor®)

All are effective, with few side effects; but each may vary somewhat in potency at certain dosages, durations of activity, and cost. All prove to be more effective when combined with healthy diets, weight reduction, exercise, and other interventions.

In addition to lowering cholesterol levels, statins also have beneficial effects on the inner surfaces of blood vessels, reducing inflammatory responses, stabilizing plaque in blood vessels, and preventing rupture of obstructing plaque, which can lead to occlusion of coronary vessels and heart attack. They also have an effect on clot formation in blood vessels.

Best of all, improvements in coronary arteries due to cholesterol reduction can occur within months of initiating treatment. Other methods of favorably effecting undesirable cholesterol levels could include hormone replacement therapy in postmenopausal women, selective estrogen-receptor modulator raloxifene (Evista®) therapy, or use of a variety of niacin preparations, which are especially helpful in raising HDL levels. Effective drug programs require close cooperation between patients and physicians, because these drugs can have serious side effects.

Lipid-lowering drug programs are usually long-term efforts. Unfortunately, about 50 percent of patients on drug programs discontinue therapy on their own within one year. Only about 25 percent of patients continue drug therapy through the end of the second year.

Recommendations

1. Know your cholesterol levels.
2. The National Cholesterol Education Program (NCEP) of the U.S. National Heart, Lung, and Blood Institute recommends that total cholesterol should be measured at least once every five years in all adults ages 20 and older. Also, if an accurate measurement is available, an HDL cholesterol level should be measured as well.
3. Know the risk factors you have and eliminate or control as many as possible.

4. Follow a regular exercise program.
5. Eat at least five servings of fruits and vegetables daily.
6. Become familiar with the American Heart Association prudent diet.
7. Middle-aged men with high cholesterol and/or other risk factors may consider having one to two alcoholic drinks daily. Alcohol intake in excess of one to two drinks per day is *not* recommended.
8. If a low-cholesterol, low-fat diet does not control your lipid problem, you may be a candidate for cholesterol-lowering drugs to be used along with your diet.
9. Follow closely the NCEP guidelines for LDL cholesterol goals as summarized below:

For individuals with:	LDL cholesterol level goals are:
Definite coronary heart disease (CHD) or other atherosclerotic disease	100 mg/dL or lower
No CHD but two or more other CHD risk factors**	130 mg/dL or lower
No CHD and fewer than two other CHD risk factors**	160 mg/dL or lower

**NCEP risk factors

NCEP risk factors are:

- Ages 45 and older in men and 55 and older in women or all women with premature menopause not using estrogen replacement therapy
- Family history of premature CHD
- Current cigarette smoking
- Hypertension (blood pressure of 140/90 mm Hg or higher) or taking antihypertensive medication
- Diabetes mellitus
- Low HDL cholesterol levels (35 mg/dL or lower) or subtract one risk factor if HDL cholesterol level is 60 mg/dL or greater

Obesity:
Benefits of and Approaches
to Weight Loss

More die in the United States of too much food than of too little.

-John Kenneth Galbraith

Facts

1. Sixty percent of adults in the U.S. are overweight, and 30 percent are obese.

2. Individuals who are 20 percent or greater over ideal body weight are at higher risk of developing coronary artery disease.

3. Individuals who are 40 percent or greater over ideal body weight are at much higher risk for cancers of the colon, prostate, breast, gallbladder, ovary, uterus, and cervix.

4. About one-third of all cases of hypertension are thought to be caused by obesity.

5. Only the Bible sells better in America than diet books.

6. The risk of diabetes increases from twofold in those who are mildly overweight to tenfold in those who are severely obese.

7. Of individuals who lose weight, up to 95 percent regain the weight in five years or less.

8. You can eat yourself to death.

9. "Apple-shaped"women are more than twice as likely to develop heart disease as are "pear-shaped" women.

Individuals who weigh 20 percent more than ideal body weight are considered obese.

Fig. 14.1 - Obesity Shape

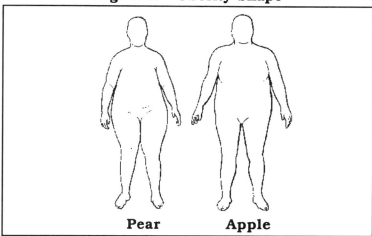

Pear   Apple

Distribution of excess weight, indicated by body shape (see Figure 14.1), is also important. Apple-shaped (top-heavy) bodies indicate that extra weight is centered around the waist; pear-shaped (bottom-heavy) bodies indicate that extra weight is centered on the hips and thighs. Of the two, apple-shaped bodies are more troublesome because they are associated with greater risks for:

- Heart disease
- Stroke
- High blood pressure
- Diabetes

Pear-shaped women are thought to have more difficulty than apple-shaped women in changing their shapes by dieting and exercise.

The size of an individual's waist can be a reflection of both total and abdominal fat. Studies suggest that waist sizes greater than 40 inches in men and 35 inches in women are associated with increased risks of acquiring a variety of significant medical problems. One study showed that women with waist measurements of 38 inches or more had greater than three times the risk of developing cardiovascular disease than those with waists of 28 inches or less.

Obesity can be found at all ages but is increasingly seen as individuals grow older and peaks at middle-age. Consideration of weight category is often viewed in relation to an individual's height (see Figure 14.2).

Fig. 14.2 - Height/Weight Chart

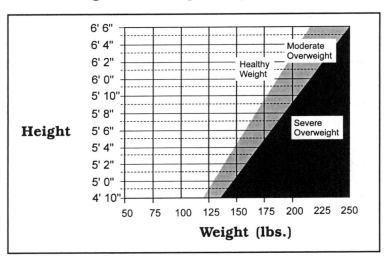

Health professionals, however, often use the Body Mass Index (BMI) (see Figure 14.3) to determine if patients are at risk. The BMI is calculated by determining a patient's weight and height and charting the findings on the BMI table; the column within which the findings are situated provides the BMI number, which serves as a reasonable estimate of fat mass.

The largest study on obesity and mortality ever conducted, involving more than one million Americans, was recently published by The American Cancer Society in The New England Journal of Medicine. It showed a definite link between being overweight and a higher risk of dying from cancer or heart disease for people of all ages. This study focused on the BMI and showed that healthy, non-smoking white men and women and black men had an increasing risk of death starting at a BMI of 25. The largest group of white males, with a BMI of 40 or greater, were found to be 2.5 times more likely to die than their healthiest peers.

This study has led researchers to suggest that obesity is probably the second leading preventable cause of death in the U.S., cigarette smoking being the first. The fact that about one-fifth of U.S. adults have a BMI of 30 or more suggests the magnitude of the problem.

The BMI number is interpreted as follows:

Underweight	Less than 18.5
Normal	18.5 to 24.9
Overweight	25 to 26.9
Obese	27 to 29.9
Moderately obese	30 to 34.9
Severely obese	35 to 39.9
Morbidly obese	Greater than 40

Fig. 14.3 – Body Mass Index

Height (inches)	Body Weight (lbs.)																
58	91	96	100	105	110	115	119	124	129	134	138	143	148	153	158	162	167
59	94	99	104	109	114	119	124	128	133	138	143	148	153	158	163	168	173
60	97	102	107	112	118	123	128	133	138	143	148	153	158	163	168	174	179
61	100	106	111	116	122	127	132	137	143	148	153	158	164	169	174	180	185
62	104	109	115	120	126	131	136	142	147	153	158	164	169	175	180	186	191
63	107	113	118	124	130	135	141	146	152	158	163	169	175	180	186	191	197
64	110	116	122	128	134	140	145	151	157	163	169	174	180	186	192	197	204
65	114	120	126	132	138	144	150	156	162	168	174	180	186	192	198	204	210
66	118	124	130	136	142	148	155	161	167	173	179	186	192	198	204	210	216
67	121	127	134	140	146	153	159	166	172	178	185	191	198	204	211	217	223
68	125	131	138	144	151	158	164	170	177	184	190	197	203	210	216	223	230
69	128	135	142	149	155	162	169	176	182	189	196	203	209	216	223	230	236
70	132	139	146	153	160	167	174	181	188	195	202	209	216	222	229	236	243
71	136	143	150	157	165	172	179	186	193	200	208	215	222	229	236	243	250
72	140	147	154	162	169	177	184	191	199	206	213	221	228	235	242	250	258
73	144	151	159	166	174	182	189	197	204	212	219	227	235	242	250	257	265
74	148	155	163	171	179	186	194	202	210	218	225	233	241	249	256	264	272
75	152	160	168	176	184	192	200	208	216	224	232	240	248	256	264	272	279
76	156	164	172	180	189	197	205	213	221	230	238	246	254	263	271	279	287
77	160	168	177	185	193	202	210	219	227	235	244	252	261	269	278	286	294
78	164	173	181	190	198	207	216	224	233	242	250	259	268	276	285	293	302
BMI =	19	20	21	22	23	24	25	26	27	28	29	30	31	32	33	34	35
	Appropriate						Overweight					Obese					

To determine BMI, locate your height in the left-hand column, then move across to your weight. Your BMI will be listed at the bottom of the column in which your height and weight intersect.

Studies suggest that up to 50 percent of those with a tendency to weight excess have some form of inherited predisposition. A recent study, however, suggests that even those with strong family histories of obesity (implying strong genetic factors that control fat mass) are still able to lose weight in response to increased physical activity, thus pointing to the importance of the behavior aspect of weight status. Other explanations for weight excess include:

- The concept that a body mechanism, possibly controlled by genes, seeks a certain weight as if it were a set point for a given individual
- Deficient exercise
- Hormonal factors
- Eating/emotional disorders (e.g., stress or depression)
- Dietary factors, such as excess fat intake

In any case, weight gain occurs when calories taken in are greater than calories expended. Every 3,500 calories consumed in excess of those burned increase weight by about one pound. The reverse is true for weight loss.

It has been estimated that the average American consumes 3,700 calories per day, though only one-half that amount for women and two-thirds that amount for men is probably needed for good body maintenance. People tend to eat more when serving sizes are larger. Our population is eating out more, where serving sizes have been getting larger in recent years. This may explain the success of certain popular and successful restaurants.

Being overweight and especially being obese have serious adverse consequences for health and longevity. Even a mild to moderate degree of weight excess can increase the risk of health complications and death at every age group.

Overweight people often have significant problems with blood fats (e.g., cholesterol and triglyceride levels), which partially explains the increased risk of coronary artery disease and likelihood of heart attack. Individuals who weigh 40 percent or more than ideal body weight are at increased risk for cancers of the:

- Colon
- Prostate
- Breast
- Gallbladder
- Kidney
- Stomach
- Uterus
- Ovary

One large study showed that women who gained more than 40 pounds after age 18 were three times more likely to have heart attacks than women who gained less than 12 pounds. Obesity is thought to be responsible for about one-third of all cases of high blood pressure.

High blood pressure in overweight people is also associated with an increased incidence of stroke and risks of developing:

- Diabetes
- Gallbladder disease
- Gout

Obesity can be associated with stresses on certain weight-bearing joints, resulting in arthritis and varying degrees of disability. Obesity, without other risk factors, may increase the likelihood of heart attack, especially for apple-shaped individuals.

In addition to known risk factors for cardiovascular disease, being of the male gender is associated with cardiovascular disease. In this regard, obesity in males is more of the apple-shape variety.

Overweight people also have more complications after surgery; wounds heal more slowly and infections are more common. Additionally, obesity is associated with:

- Anxiety
- Stress
- Depression
- Sleep disturbances (sleep apnea)
- Other consequences that affect quality and length of life

For improvement in quality and length of life, overweight and obese individuals should strive to achieve weights that are close to ideal for their ages, genders, heights, and body builds. A recent large study of nurses has put to rest concerns about adverse effects of thinness. That study showed that increased death rates thought to be present in very thin people were partly due to cigarette smoking or weight loss associated with cancers or other serious conditions.

It may be impossible for some individuals to reach desired weights, but even modest weight reduction has been associated with increased longevity and improved diabetes and high blood pressure control. It has been suggested that the initial goal of weight loss therapy should be to reduce body weight by approximately 10 percent from the initial weight. The need or desirability of further weight loss can then be considered. To achieve this first weight loss, patients should structure a caloric deficit of about 500 to 1,000 calories per day, mostly by eating less. Some of the deficit, possibly 20 percent, could be derived from a modest, daily exercise program. Weight reduction can be achieved with the help of a physician or by the team approach of a physician, dietitian, and counselor.

Dieting alone can help weight loss, but exercise provides additional benefits. Regular physical activity is especially important for weight maintenance. Exercise alone, however, is a difficult way to lose pounds. It has been suggested that one would have to walk or run 35 miles to lose one pound. Exercise is helpful in preventing one from regaining lost weight. Physicians or psychiatrists/psychologists can assist with behavior modification programs.

Also, certain drugs can help in special situations. Physician-prescribed appetite suppressants, always combined with prudent diets, can provide superior weight loss results compared with diet therapy alone. However, some diet medications have significant side effects, including an extremely rare form of irreversible high blood pressure in the pulmonary vessels. These medications should be used only under the direction of physicians.

Older amphetamine-based appetite suppressants are rarely used today. Another group of appetite suppressants was recently withdrawn from the market because of drug associations with cardiac valve problems. A newer drug, sibutramine (Meridia®), affects the brain chemicals that help control appetite. Though not shown to cause heart valve problems, this agent can raise blood pressure levels in some individuals. It can be useful for significantly obese individuals whose serious health problems from their obesity outweigh the risks of taking the medicine. As with all antiobesity agents, patients must be closely monitored.

The newest antiobesity drug on the U.S. market is orlistat (Xenical®), which acts by inhibiting absorption from the gut of about 30 percent of the fat that is ingested. Studies suggest that this drug causes modest weight loss and certain health benefits related to that loss. An advantage of this agent over others is the fact that less than one percent of the drug passes from the bowel into the blood, making it less likely to cause side effects in other organs of the body. Problems related to Xenical® have been largely centered in the gastrointestinal tract and are due to the increased fat in the stool. The drug's mechanism of action can affect blood levels of fat-soluble vitamins such as A and E; thus, vitamin supplements are needed with this therapy. Long-term adverse effects of prolonged use are as yet unknown.

Pregnant women and individuals ages 65 and older should not initiate diets without consulting their physicians. For the severely obese patient (weight at 100 percent or 100 lbs. above ideal) who is at high risk for adverse health problems related to the obesity, surgery appears to be a reasonable option. Various surgical procedures, performed by skilled surgeons at specialized referral centers, offer the best long-term hope for these individuals. Patients undergoing such procedures must be followed for extended periods postoperatively to avoid potential complications. For certain individuals, weight-loss surgery results in impressive improvement in weight and health. Over a one- to two-year period after such surgery, an individual can lose 50 to 60 percent of the excess weight.

Liposuction cannot be recommended for such patients because the fatty tissue removed has been known to reaccumulate in the same site or at times at other sites.

The American public is deluged with dietary advice in the forms of books, tapes, and videos. In many cases, the advice is wrong, unsound, unhealthy, and dangerous. Though it would be impossible to comment on all the dietary plans available, the authors suggest that patients would do best by avoiding presently popular plans suggested in Dr. Atkins' New Diet Revolution, The Five Day Miracle Diet, The Beverly Hills Diet, Sugar Busters!, Enter the Zone, and Protein Power. Before embarking on any new diet program, patients should check with their physicians or with registered dietitians for advice. Another option is to seek help from weight-loss organizations such as Weight Watchers, TOPS, Jenny Craig, and other organizations that have joined the Federal Trade Commission's Partnership for Healthy Weight Management.

Use of alternative medicine approaches to weight loss have become popular in recent years. Such products as chromium picolinate, ma huang, hydroxycitric acid found in plants, Garcinia cambogia, and Garcinia indica, to name but a few, have not been proven effective; and at times some have been proven to be toxic. These are best avoided.

Recommendations

1. Try to achieve a weight close to ideal for your age, sex, build, height, and musculature.
2. Dieting, as suggested by your physician, and exercise should be the basis of any weight-loss program. This will work even if you have inherited a tendency toward obesity.
3. If you are unable to achieve ideal weight, lose as much weight as you can.
4. Avoid fad diets and medications or programs not approved by your physician.
5. Before initiating any weight loss program, determine if you have a medical condition (e.g., hypothyroidism, adrenal hormone excess, Cushing's syndrome, or kidney, heart, or liver disease) that causes weight gain or if you take medications that contribute to weight gain (e.g., cortisone preparations).

Alcohol: Do Benefits Outweigh Dangers?

Eat not to dullness. Drink not to elevation.

-Benjamin Franklin

Facts

1. Alcohol-related deaths account for 2.7 million patient years of potential life lost annually in the U.S.; 65 percent of that loss is due to alcohol-related injuries.

2. People dying from alcohol-related causes lose an average of 26 years of normal life expectancy.

3. About one-third of drivers killed in vehicle crashes are intoxicated by alcohol.

4. The risk of dying in a traffic accident is eight times greater for heavy drinkers than for nondrinkers.

5. The risk of fatal single-vehicle crashes in drivers with blood alcohol concentrations of 0.09 percent (less than the common standard for driving legally, 0.10 percent) is 11.1 times greater than for nondrinkers. At blood alcohol concentrations of 0.15 percent or greater, the risk is 380 times greater.

6. Of suicide victims, 50 percent are intoxicated with alcohol or other drugs.

7. It appears that, in women, two to three drinks per day is associated with a 30-percent increase in breast cancer incidence or mortality; higher levels of alcohol consumption are associated with a 70-percent increase.

Alcohol is believed to be the most frequently abused drug throughout the world. It is associated with shortening life, as a prominent contributor to:

❂ Death and debility from automobile accidents
❂ Suicides
❂ Other violent deaths

In the U.S. about 100,000 deaths each year are attributed to alcohol. Additionally, liver cirrhosis, often a complication of alcoholism, is a relatively common cause of death among individuals ages 25 to 46. The presence of cirrhosis caused by alcohol considerably shortens the expected lifespan. Significant alcohol ingestion over many years can result in severe heart problems and heart failure; short-term heavy ingestion, such as with binge drinking, can lead to heart rhythm disturbances and even death.

Alcohol abuse also has been linked with cancers of the gastrointestinal and respiratory tracts and even the breast. Women who drink similar amounts as men appear to be at greater risk for complications because they:

❂ Appear to metabolize alcohol differently from men
❂ Have a lower volume of body water
❂ Reach a higher blood alcohol concentration in a shorter period of time with the same intake

Moderate drinking is defined as two drinks per day for men and one per day for women (a drink equals 12 oz. of regular beer, 5 oz. wine, or 1½ oz. of distilled spirits at 80-percent proof). One study found that ingestion of more than two drinks per day and progressively greater levels of consumption were associated with higher all-cause mortality.

It has become apparent that moderate to heavy drinkers (i.e., those who drink three or more alcoholic beverages per day) have an increased risk of liver damage and stomach bleeding when taking aspirin, other salicylates, acetaminophen, ibuprofen, naproxen, or ketoprofen, medicines recognized as over-the-counter pain relievers and fever reducers.

Alcohol is also a problem for the elderly. Up to 10 percent of older adults living at home may have problems with alcohol, and an even greater problem is seen in nursing homes.

Because their body fluids are decreased, the elderly who drink have resulting higher rates of blood alcohol levels and complications than younger people who drink the same amount of alcohol. Alcohol excess in the elderly can lead to various other problems, such as:

○ Blood pressure elevation
○ Depression
○ Frequent falls
○ Nutritional, vitamin, and mineral deficiencies
○ Degenerative brain disorders
○ Dementia

Because older adults often live alone, their drinking problems may not be recognized until major problems develop and mortality is high. Professional help is important in this group, whose responses to treatment are as good as those of younger drinkers.

Those who drink alcoholic beverages must determine their limitations of alcohol intake and maintain control of intake. Help in determining personal alcohol dependence can be obtained from answers to the CAGE questionnaire:

C - Have you considered **C**utting down on your drinking?

A - Have you ever become **A**ngry or **A**nnoyed about questions concerning your drinking?

G - Have you ever felt **G**uilty about your drinking practices?

E - Do you ever begin your day with an **E**ye opener?

A result of two or more "yes" answers to the questionnaire suggests the likelihood of alcohol dependence; a result of "yes" answers to all four strongly points to it. The recognition of alcohol dependence should be followed by treatment programs organized by personal physicians or special teams with recognized expertise.

People with family histories of alcoholism are at risk of becoming alcoholics themselves. In fact, drinkers with alcoholic parents are four times more likely to have problems with alcohol consumption than drinkers who have no family histories of alcohol problems. Genes have a lot to do with our risks of becoming alcohol-dependent but are not exclusive predictors of such risk. Environmental factors (e.g., adverse life events or work-related stresses) are also important.

The earlier that alcohol dependence is detected and treated, the more likely that it can be successfully treated and complications (e.g., liver, heart, and neurological disorders) can be avoided. As many as 50 percent of alcohol-dependent individuals do not recognize their disorder.

At present, there is no universally effective approach to the treatment of alcohol dependence; a variety of psychological, social, and medical interventions have proved effective to one degree or another. In combination with these interventions, certain drug therapies can improve outcomes. An older drug, disulfiram (Antabuse®), deters alcohol ingestion by triggering adverse reactions (e.g., nausea, vomiting, diarrhea, and flushing) in those who imbibe. Though potentially effective, this drug has been associated with significant problems and is not frequently used at this time. A newer drug, naltrexone (ReVia®), has been effective in reducing alcohol consumption and increasing abstinence by lessening the pleasurable effects of alcohol and reducing cravings for it; this effect occurs in alcoholic patients as well as in social drinkers. The drug is especially useful when combined with other therapeutic interventions. Other drugs not yet available in the U.S. appear promising.

Another facet of alcohol ingestion must also be considered in view of recent findings. It appears that moderate consumption of alcohol (no more than two standard drinks daily for men and one for women) may be a reasonably good thing. Studies suggest that this consumption exerts a protective effect against coronary artery disease. Consuming one or two alcoholic drinks daily results in a 30- to 60-percent reduction in the risk of developing coronary artery disease and even appears to improve the chances of survival should a heart attack develop.

The mechanism for this beneficial effect could be the ability of alcohol to elevate HDL cholesterol. Much has been written about the type of alcohol that is most beneficial. In several regions of France, its populace eats diets that are rich in saturated fats and cholesterol, yet the country boasts a low incidence of coronary artery disease, a situation termed as the French Paradox.

Some researchers suggest that it is red wine, popular in France, that provides protection because it, unlike white wine, incorporates the skins of red grapes (which contain large amounts of phenolic compounds that behave like antioxidants) into the production process. Antioxidants, along with other substances in red wine that prevent blood clotting, may explain the reduction in coronary risk.

Other researchers believe that ethanol itself causes the beneficial effect, which then could explain similar benefits from ingesting red or white wine, beer, or other spirits. Many believe that other factors common to the French should also be considered, such as the increased amounts of fruits and vegetables (containing antioxidant vitamins) this group consumes or the fact that the French drink alcohol in moderation and with meals. Also, these groups dine differently than Americans, eating more heavily at midday than in the evening.

Other elements of the French or Mediterranean diet, e.g., eating olive oil and garlic, may also be important. Still other explanations for the French paradox have been suggested. The French may not classify all the same entities recognized by the Americans and British as causes of death from coronary artery disease. Additionally, it has been suggested that the French people have not had a long enough exposure to the high animal fat diets they presently consume to have manifested the consequences of these diets, as are seen in other Western countries. It must be remembered, however, that the French, who boast the largest consumption of wine in the world, have much higher rates than other groups with lesser alcohol intakes of:

- Cirrhosis
- Upper gastrointestinal malignancies
- Accidents
- Suicides
- Violent deaths

Alcohol in moderation (i.e., one to two drinks daily) appears to lower risks for ischemic stroke, the most common type, which usually results from the development of a blood clot in an atherosclerotic blood vessel that supplies a portion of the brain. All forms of alcoholic beverages are beneficial in the modest consumptions suggested, but larger amounts (seven or more drinks daily) significantly increases risks of this stroke type. Though the exact mechanism for this protective effect with alcohol is not known, several factors, no doubt, contribute, such as alcohol's ability to increase HDL cholesterol levels and to interfere with clot formation in cerebral and coronary arteries.

Recommendations
1. If you don't drink, don't start.
2. If you wish to drink, some cardiac benefits may be derived from light to moderate drinking of:
   - No more than two drinks daily for men
   - No more than one drink daily for women
   - No more than one drink daily for those ages 65 and older

3. Discuss openly your alcohol intake with your physician.
4. Individuals with concerns about breast or gastrointestinal cancers or strong family histories of alcoholism should discuss these situations with their physicians.
5. Some people should consider avoiding alcohol altogether, including:
   - Women who are pregnant or are trying to conceive
   - People who plan to drive or perform other activities that require unimpaired attention or muscular coordination
   - Individuals taking antihistamines, sedatives, or other medications that can magnify alcohol's effects
   - Recovering alcoholics
   - Persons being treated for anxiety or depression, since alcohol is thought to affect their clinical course and response to treatment

Further Reading

Ewing JA: Detecting alcoholism: The CAGE questionnaire. JAMA 1984;252:1905-1907.

Stress and Depression: Avoidance and Treatment as Paths to Happiness

A vigorous five-mile walk will do more good for an unhappy but otherwise healthy adult than all the medicine and psychology in the world.

-Paul Dudley White

Facts

1. Primary care physicians treat depression and anxiety more than they treat heart disease, hypertension, or diabetes.

2. Up to 50 percent of patients with unexplained chest pains are really suffering from anxiety.

3. One-third of coronary artery patients have disease-related depression or anxiety.

4. About 25 percent of all suicides are committed by individuals ages 60 and older.

5. Depressed persons have suicide rates at least eight times higher than those of the general population.

6. Psychosocial stress interventions (i.e., group psychotherapy, counseling, relaxation training, and stress-reduction programs) reduce recurrent cardiac events (e.g., death and heart attacks) by 35 to 75 percent.

7. Pet owners have fewer risk factors for heart disease than individuals without such companions.

8. Depressed people have increased mortality from coronary artery disease and cancer.

9. Depression is common in smokers and those who are alcohol-dependent.

10. Up to two-thirds of persons with depression go undetected and untreated.

11. Depressive disorders occur in an estimated six percent of the general population but may be found in as many as 50 percent of those with medical illnesses.

At many points in life, individuals face various stresses of varying degrees. Such stresses can aggravate existing medical problems and possibly trigger new conditions. Various stressors have at times been associated with increased risks for heart attacks or strokes; these include:

- Anger
- Death of someone close
- Involvement in a war
- Being present during an earthquake or other catastrophe

Other stresses, especially when problems are ongoing, may lead to various problems, from high blood pressure to cancer to sudden death; such stresses include:

- Major financial problems
- Significant family problems
- Loss of loved ones
- Unresolved grief
- Occupational stress
- Divorce
- Having certain diseases or physical problems

These responses to stresses and/or their complications can be associated with shortened lifespans. Stressful life events themselves can significantly increase risks of death; such events include:

- Divorce or separation
- Financial difficulty
- Being sued
- Insecure feelings at work

One interesting study shows that the risk of heart attack increases 14-fold in the first 24 hours after the death of a loved one. By the end of the second day, the risk was still eight times higher than normal.

People who have family histories of depression or live particularly stressful lives are also prone to depression, especially if they:

- Have sudden, major life changes
- Are unmarried or widowed
- Lack supportive social networks
- Have certain physical conditions, such as:
  - Cancer
  - Stroke
  - Heart disease
  - Dementia
  - Any chronic illness

One study has shown that death occurs several times more frequently in heart attack patients who also meet criteria for major depression in the six months after the event than those without depression. It also appears that the recent development of depression (not chronic depression) in older men is a risk factor for heart attacks.

Depression is also associated with biochemical disruptions in the brain, which fortunately respond to drug treatment. Drug treatment can also be effective in treating depression that results from stressful events.

Depression is common in American society, with about 15 percent of the population suffering from a major depressive disorder at some time in their lives. Unfortunately, this disorder is diagnosed and treated in less than one-third of these individuals.

Among the elderly, major or minor depression is seen in about five percent of patients in primary care clinics and up to 25 percent of patients in nursing homes. Sadly, most elderly people with depression fail to seek help. Moreover, depression can mimic dementia in the elderly.

Depressed individuals often have repeated visits to their physicians with complaints of:
- Vague pain
- Low energy
- Fatigue
- Insomnia
- Digestive problems
- Sexual difficulties

Physicians often fail to recognize symptoms of depression, which include:
- Persistent feelings of:
  - Sadness
  - Hopelessness
  - Pessimism
  - Anxiety
- Loss of interest or pleasure in ordinary activities, including sex
- Irritability
- Restlessness
- Decreased energy
- Fatigue
- Feeling slowed down
- Loss of appetite
- Weight loss
- Unintentional weight gain
- Sleeping too little or too much
- Difficulty with:
  - Concentration
  - Remembering
  - Making decisions

- Feelings of:
  - Guilt
  - Worthlessness
  - Helplessness
- Thoughts of death or suicide
- Suicide attempts
- Not caring whether one lives or dies from medical illness
- Excessive crying
- Recurrent aches and pains that do not respond to treatment
- Personality change
- Substance abuse

Of concern for all patients with depression is the possibility of suicide. Depression appears to be associated with about one-half of all suicides and is one of the strongest factors for attempted and completed suicides.

Suicide is a special problem in depressed older adults. About 25 percent of all suicides are committed by individuals ages 60 and older.

Depression is often a recurrent illness, but it can be treated effectively if it is recognized. Certain illicit drugs, alcohol, and prescription and nonprescription medicines can cause or complicate depression. Depression may also be a side effect of various medications or may be associated with numerous medical illnesses. Depression can also be related to seasonal decreases in the length of daylight, noted at both the northern and southern latitudes.

It has become clear that isolation from others is detrimental. Though data on the value of human connections are difficult to obtain, it appears that people with adequate social networks suffer less depression and live longer than those without such support systems. Valuable support system assets that allow and help people cope with stresses and complexities of life include:

- Friends
- Companions
- Acquaintances
- Comrades
- Spouses
- Associates
- Lovers
- Families
- Pets

Of untold value is belonging to such groups as:

- Religious communities
- Social networks
- Families
- Communities
- Sports teams

Fortunately, medications are available that are safe and effective for the treatment of depression. Drug therapy, in fact, is the first-line treatment for depression.

A variety of effective antidepressants are available; these include:

- Selective serotonin re-uptake inhibitors (SSRIs)
- Tricyclics
- Tetracyclics
- Lithium

Drugs from these groups when combined with psychotherapy may be even more effective. These drugs can be effective within weeks, allowing the depressed individual to return to normal daily activities rather quickly. Continued therapy is effective in preventing recurrent bouts of depression.

Electroconvulsive therapy is occasionally used and is effective for cases of severe depression. It is suggested that 80 percent of people with serious depression will improve with medications and/or psychological counseling.

Recommendations
1. Do not be afraid to ask for help.
2. If you can eliminate, reduce, or modify stresses in your life, do so. Discussion of your stresses with physicians, psychiatrists/psychologists, or friends may help.
3. A routine exercise program often proves valuable for a variety of mental and emotional problems.
4. Maintain regular hours of adequate sleep (six to eight hours daily).
5. If you have symptoms of depression, seek your physician's help to sort out possible causes (e.g., drugs, illnesses) and start you on a treatment program.
6. Although thoughts of suicide are common in depression, such thoughts should encourage prompt consultation with your physician.
7. Develop and foster support groups in your life.
8. Do not drink alcohol if you are depressed or anxious or caffeine beverages if you are anxious; such drinks may increase symptoms.

Immunizations: Increased Means of Disease Prevention

The value of life lies not in the length of days, but in the use we make of them. A man may live long yet live very little.

-Montaigne

Facts

1. Each year in the U.S., influenza, pneumococcal disease, and hepatitis kill 50,000 to 90,000 adults.

2. Among older adults, only 52 percent receive influenza vaccines and 28 percent receive pneumococcal vaccines. These vaccines are free to Medicare and Medicaid beneficiaries.

3. Vaccines in adults can prevent 70 percent of deaths due to influenza, 60 percent of cases of invasive pneumococcal disease, and 90 percent of hepatitis cases.

4. Influenza is one of the leading causes of death in people older than age 65 and is the most common infectious cause of death in the U.S.

5. Less than one-third of the high-risk persons for whom influenza immunization is recommended have received the vaccine.

6. An estimated 40,000 lives would be saved each year in the U.S. if vaccines against influenza, pneumococcus, and hepatitis B virus were beneficially employed.

Immunizations can reduce the incidence of major causes of disease, disability, and death in adults, especially in older populations. Routine vaccination programs can save lives with minimal effort expended.

INFLUENZA VACCINE

Most deaths from influenza virus infections occur in the elderly. In the U.S., 10,000 to 50,000 deaths each year have been associated with various epidemics. Vaccination from influenza results in:
◉ Less severe illness
◉ Lower fever
◉ Lower medical expenses
◉ Considerably lowered mortality

The U.S. Public Health Service recommends that influenza vaccines be given to all persons ages 65 and older as well as to younger persons in certain high-risk groups, including:
◉ Residents of chronic care facilities
◉ Individuals who suffer from chronic heart or lung disorders
◉ Individuals with chronic metabolic diseases, such as:
  ◉ Diabetes mellitus
  ◉ Kidney dysfunction
  ◉ Blood diseases
  ◉ Lowered body immune resistance
◉ Individuals who travel to developing countries where medical care is less than optimal

Studies among groups most likely to benefit found that influenza vaccinations can reduce the number of cases of influenza by at least 70 percent, the number of hospital admissions for influenza-related pneumonia by 45 percent, and influenza-related deaths by 40 percent. Studies have shown that as many as 10 to 15 persons are hospitalized for each person who dies of complications from influenza. Influenza immunizations significantly reduce risks of hospitalization of elderly patients.

Vaccination of the staff in geriatric centers is important and can reduce the mortality from influenza among patients in such facilities.

For individuals at high risk who have not received the influenza vaccine at the time of an outbreak, two drugs, amantadine (Symmetrel®) and rimantadine (Flumadine®) are very effective in preventing influenza A when given for 10 days after exposure. These drugs can also be used in the treatment of influenza in individuals at high risk. They should be started within 48 hours of the onset of symptoms. Two new drugs that can be used to treat influenza A or B or provide prophylaxis in nursing homes or among families (zanamivir [Relenza™] and oseltamivir [Tamiflu™]) are noted in Chapter 8.

PNEUMOCOCCAL VACCINE

Pneumococcal disease causes about 40,000 deaths, 500,000 cases of pneumonia, and 50,000 cases of bacteremia (bacteria present in circulating blood) each year in the U.S. It also causes about 3,000 cases of meningitis and about seven million ear infections yearly. Mortality rates are highest among the elderly and those with chronic diseases.

In spite of these facts, only 30 percent of persons older than age 65 receive the pneumococcal vaccine. The pneumococcal vaccine is recommended for all adults who are 65 years and older and for adults younger than age 65 who have a variety of chronic illnesses. Recent studies have also shown that the pneumococcus bacteria is the most common organism found in patients with community-acquired pneumonia. Because of this prevalence and the recognition of increased resistance of this organism to commonly prescribed antibiotics, more aggressive vaccine programs to prevent pneumococcal pneumonia would appear to be desirable.

The efficacy of the pneumococcal vaccine varies depending on the groups evaluated but is about 60 percent or greater in most patient groups. Though it may not always prevent a pneumonia, its major benefit has been in preventing more serious cases and death. It is thought that the vaccine has the potential to prevent half of pneumococcal disease deaths in the U.S.

The incidence of pneumococcal pneumonia is higher in:

- Nursing home residents
- Alcoholics
- Individuals with certain chronic medical conditions
- Jail or prison inmates
- Patients with absent or nonfunctioning spleens

TETANUS VACCINE

In the U.S., tetanus, though rare, has become a disease of the elderly, with more than 50 percent of cases occurring in adults ages 60 and older and most deaths occurring in patients ages 40 and older. Tetanus is found in individuals who have never received completed vaccination series as a children. About 30 to 60 percent of adults ages 60 and older lack protective levels of tetanus antibodies. Death occurs in up to 24 percent of tetanus cases, with mortality being highest in the elderly.

Tetanus vaccination is effective.

Although diphtheria is rare in the U.S., it is increasing in other countries; thus, the diphtheria vaccine is given along with tetanus.

HEPATITIS B VACCINE

Up to 300,000 individuals become infected with hepatitis B virus in the U.S. each year. Some of these individuals develop chronic active hepatitis and even cirrhosis. Complications of hepatitis B infection result in about 5,000 deaths per year in the U.S.

Hepatitis B is transmitted from person to person. The group at highest risk is intravenous drug users and their sex partners. Other high-risk groups include:

- Men who have sex with men
- Those with histories of sexual activities with multiple partners
- Travelers to high-risk areas
- Persons in health-related jobs who are exposed to blood or blood products
- Dialysis patients

The hepatitis B virus is transmitted through body fluids such as vaginal secretions, semen, and blood. It can survive outside the body for up to one month, however; thus, there is potential for infection from items like toothbrushes, razors, unsterilized manicure instruments, and electrolysis needles that have been in contact with infected body fluids.

The hepatitis B vaccine has proven to be effective.

HEPATITIS A VACCINE

Epidemics of hepatitis A are usually caused by fecally contaminated water or food; this situation is responsible for about one-half of cases in the U.S., at least 27,000 cases each year.

A certain small mortality is associated with hepatitis A, but mortality increases with increasing age. Certain individuals are at higher risk for hepatitis A, including:

- Institutionalized persons and workers at such institutions
- Travelers to countries where hepatitis A is common
- Men who have sex with men
- Users of injection or street drugs
- Those in close contact with hepatitis A persons

The effectiveness of the hepatitis A vaccine appears to be quite good.

LYME DISEASE VACCINE

Lyme disease is the most common insect-transmitted disease in the U.S. and has the potential to develop serious rheumatic, neurological, and cardiac complications. It is found only in certain areas of the U.S. Thus, the Lyme disease vaccine should be considered for persons who reside, work, or play in areas of high or moderate risk during the transmission season. The vaccine is about 76-percent effective after three doses but is much more effective in protecting against asymptomatic disease.

VARICELLA

Chicken pox tends to be more severe in adults and patients with immune deficiencies, causing increased complications, such as encephalitis, in those groups. About five percent of adults in the U.S. are susceptible to varicella.

Vaccination is effective, protecting 95 percent of recipients from getting a serious form of the disease.

Recommendations

1. Obtain the necessary immunizations at appropriate ages, and keep immunizations current.
2. Travelers to third world countries should consider having hepatitis vaccines.

Further Reading

Guide to Clinical Preventive Services, Report of the U.S. Preventive Services Task Force, 2nd ed. Williams & Wilkins 1996.

Diet:
The Benefits of Fresh Fruits and Vegetables

One should eat to live, not live to eat.

-Moliére

Facts

1. Studies suggest that reducing dietary fat to less than 30 percent of total calories can lower coronary artery disease mortality rates by as much as 20 percent.

2. Only about 20 percent of the U.S. population achieves the desired goal of 30 percent or less of calories from fat.

3. The average American's diet is 36 percent fat.

4. It is estimated that up to 50 percent of nursing home residents in the U.S. may be malnourished.

5. A large study of British subjects showed that daily consumption of fresh fruit was associated with significantly fewer deaths from coronary artery disease and stroke.

6. Though not generally known or recognized, trans-fatty acids (produced by a manufacturing process that adds hydrogen atoms to unsaturated fats to make them more saturated and thus more solid) may be more harmful than saturated fats.

What we eat, how much we eat, and what we don't eat has important consequences to the quality and length of our lives. It is important that we establish healthy dietary patterns as early in life as possible and that we maintain these patterns throughout life.

What is eaten influences the development of such problems as:

○ High blood pressure
○ Coronary artery disease
○ Stroke
○ Several different cancers
○ Type 2 diabetes
○ Gallbladder disease

Recent studies have shown that lowering cholesterol in the blood through drug therapy in people with histories of coronary artery disease or prior heart attack and elevated cholesterol levels definitely lengthened life. In this group, the risk of death from heart disease was 42 percent lower than for those untreated.

Earlier studies by researchers such as Dean Ornish showed that coronary artery disease progression could be arrested and even reversed through programs of:

○ Diet
○ Exercise
○ Stress reduction

Dr. Ornish currently is conducting a large multicenter study to confirm these observations. The Ornish diet program is rigorous but effective. It restricts fat intake to less than 10 percent of total calories, excluding all oils and animal products except for nonfat yogurt, skim milk, and egg whites. The program allows only 5 to 10 mg of dietary cholesterol daily.

This regimen contrasts with the American Heart Association program, which recommends no more than 30 percent of total calories from fat and daily cholesterol intake of less than 300 mg (one egg has about 215 mg of cholesterol).

A recent study from the Cleveland Clinic, also based on a diet with less than 10 percent calories from fat, along with use of cholesterol-lowering medications, proved effective in stopping the progression of coronary artery disease over many years. These impressive results were achieved without the meditation, stress management, and lifestyle changes featured in the Ornish program.

Many experts believe that the regimen of 30 percent of total calories as dietary fat is too high and that 20 to 25 percent is a more prudent figure. At present, the typical American diet is greater than 36 percent fat, a level that is sure to cause health problems for certain individuals.

Excessive reduction of total fat intake and subsequent replacement with carbohydrates can also cause problems, namely the reduction of protective HDL cholesterol levels and elevated triglyceride levels. Drastic reductions of fatty foods could also deprive the body of certain necessary nutrients and create difficulty in the body's ability to absorb essential fat-soluble vitamins.

A prudent diet for most individuals is the dietary program endorsed by the American Heart

Association (see Recommendations). Lack of response to that diet or lack of motivation to achieve better results with diet might make Dr. Ornish's program appealing. In any case, working with physicians and registered dietitians provides the best opportunity to find diets that are healthful and easy to follow.

At present, only about 20 percent of the U.S. population achieves the average daily goal of no more than 30 percent of calories from fat. Great importance should be attached to the amounts and types of fat in the diet. Dietary fats are classified as saturated or unsaturated. Saturated fats are the most powerful dietary contributors to high blood cholesterol levels, particularly raising LDL blood levels. These fats present a special problem because they interfere with removal of cholesterol from the blood, which in turn results in elevation of blood cholesterol. The body gets along nicely without saturated fats in the diet because of its ability to produce them.

Trans-fatty acids are formed when manufacturers' process foods to make their unsaturated fats more solid and shelf-stable (e.g., margarine). These foods then have the LDL cholesterol-elevating ability of saturated fats but may also lower HDL cholesterol levels and even increase triglyceride levels, making them more potentially harmful than saturated fatty acids. Many fast foods (e.g., doughnuts and French fries) have high levels of trans-fatty acids, which are not required to be listed on food labels.

Unsaturated fats, found primarily in plants, are of two kinds: monounsaturated and polyunsaturated. When substituted for saturated fats in the diet, these fats can actually be associated with reducing LDL cholesterol levels.

Examples of dietary fats are:

SATURATED	MONOUNSATURATED	POLYUNSATURATED
Butter	Avocado	Corn oil
Cheese	Canola oil	Cottonseed oil
Chocolate	Cashews	Margarine
Cocoa butter	Olives	Mayonnaise
Coconut	Olive oil	Pecans
Cream	Peanuts	Safflower oil
Egg yoke	Peanut butter	Soybean oil
Hydrogenated oil	Macadamia nuts	Sunflower seeds
Lard	Hazelnuts	Walnuts
Meat	Pistachios	Pine nuts
Poultry		Almonds

Monounsaturated fatty acids are more desirable than the polyunsaturated variety because they are more difficult to oxidize, a process that contributes to plaque formation in arterial walls. However, too much unsaturated fat of either variety can also increase risks of heart disease and cancer.

Some individuals find it difficult to follow diet programs and resist formal programs proposed for them. In such cases, it may be better for physicians to provide basic eating guidelines, which may include suggestions that patients:

- Maintain desirable or ideal weights for their heights
- Eat less fat, especially animal fat and cholesterol
- Eat less meat

○ Eat more plant foods, at least five portions of fruits and vegetables each day; several studies have shown that individuals who eat large amounts of fruits and vegetables have lower risks of developing:
  ○ High blood pressure
  ○ Several cancers
  ○ Strokes (see Chapter 3)

A significant decrease in heart attack risks occurs as the amount of fiber in the diet is increased. Fiber, the indigestible component of plant foods, can be found in:
○ Fruits and vegetables
○ Whole grains
○ Beans
○ Nuts
○ Seeds
○ Breads
○ Pastas

Whole grains are much more valuable than refined grains because they have higher fiber contents, more nutrients, and more valuable phytochemicals with antioxidant capabilities. Sources of insoluble fiber include whole-grain cereals, whole-wheat bread, and crackers. Soluble fiber, found in legumes, fruits, oats, barley, and some vegetables, is capable of lowering cholesterol levels. High-fiber foods are also valuable because they tend to be filling. Studies suggest that fiber may reduce calorie intake by blocking the digestion (absorption) of fats and proteins eaten with it.

Unfortunately, most people get only 15 grams of the 25 to 30 grams of fiber considered to be desirable in the daily diet. A variety of foods and supplements with high-fiber content include:

Post 100% Bran® (1/3 cup) .... 8 g
Kellogg's Rasin Bran® (1 cup) .... 8 g
Kellogg's All-Bran Extra Fiber® (1/2 cup) .... 13 g
General Mills Fiber One® (1/2 cup) .... 13 g
Apple (medium with skin) .... 3.7 g
Avocado (one medium) .... 8.5 g
Prunes (10, dried) .... 6 g
Kidney beans, red (1 cup, boiled) .... 13 g
Lima beans (1/2 cup) .... 6.6 g
Metamucil® (1 rounded tsp.) .... 3.4 g
Perdiem®, plain (1 rounded tsp.) .... 4 g
Citrucel® (1 rounded tsp.) .... 2 g

The U.S. Department of Agriculture recommends a diet program based on numbers of servings each day (based on caloric intake) from each of five food groups (see Figure 18.1). In the guide, the lower number of recommended servings is for the equivalent of a 1,600-calorie diet and the upper number for a 2,800-calorie diet.

Fig. 18.1 - Food Guide Pyramid

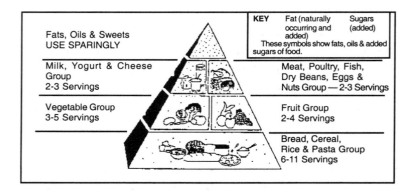

The pyramid is an outline of what to eat each day rather than a rigid prescription. It calls for eating a variety of foods in order to receive needed nutrients. Foods in one group cannot replace those in another. The base of the pyramid suggests foods that should be the major components of our diets. As we move up the pyramid, we move in the direction of foods we should eat less often. At the top are the foods that should be used sparingly.

A similar pyramid could be constructed for the so-called Mediterranean diet, which contains much less red meat, plenty of fruits and vegetables, olive oil as the main source of fat, plant proteins as the major source of protein, and moderate wine consumption. Recent studies of such a diet from Lyon, France, however, made it apparent how similar it is, with regard to fat content, to the American Heart Association diet.

A pyramid constructed for a healthy Asian diet would also de-emphasize red meat, emphasize plant foods (especially rice), and feature vegetable oils in place of olive oils. A pyramid constructed for elderly individuals would emphasize adequate fluid intake (at least eight glasses of water, juice, or milk), more fiber, and greater amounts of vitamins B_{12} and D.

In all diets, eating a fatty fish (e.g., salmon, mackerel, herring, sardines, or tuna) even once per week has been associated with a reduced risk of coronary artery disease, possibly related to the omega-3 fatty acids present in fish oils. Fish oils are known to reduce triglyceride levels in people with prominent hypertriglyceridemia. The addition of 1 gram of omega-3 fish oil supplement to a good diet has also proven effective after a heart attack.

Fruits and vegetables are loaded with micronutrients, including vitamins, minerals, antioxidants, disease-preventing phytochemicals, disease-preventing or disease-fighting indoles, isothiocynates, sulforaphane, phenic acids, potential estrogen-like compounds known as phytoestrogens, infection-fighting saponins, and fiber.

The value of fruits and vegetables in the diet is becoming more apparent; not only are these foods helpful in avoiding coronary artery disease, but they also have a place in cancer prevention. The National Cancer Institute supports a program that includes eating five or more servings of fruits and vegetables each day as part of a low-fat, high-fiber diet. Certain nutrients (carotenoids) found in fruits and vegetables have been shown to lower risks of developing age-related macular degeneration, the most important cause of irreversible blindness among those 65 years and older.

Studies show that less than one-third of the population actually achieves this goal and that the majority of people consume less than one serving of fruit per day. Worse yet, only about one-fourth of the population is aware of this dietary recommendation.

Some people are confused by the recommendations for fruits and vegetables. A recent *British Medical Journal* article helps clarify some of these concerns. The authors recommend eating a wide variety of fruits and vegetables, allowing in this

category the inclusion of such items as:
- ⚙ Fruit juice
- ⚙ Baked beans
- ⚙ Dried fruit
- ⚙ Frozen and canned fruit
- ⚙ Vegetables and fruits as found in pies

They exclude:
- ⚙ Potatoes
- ⚙ Fruit drinks
- ⚙ Nuts

The article also clarifies the meaning of a serving or portion in a way that is more readily understood:

FOOD TYPE	PORTION (Serving)*	EXAMPLE
FRUITS		
Very large fruit	One large slice	Melon, pineapple
Large fruit	One whole	Apple, banana
Medium fruit	Two whole	Plum, kiwi
Berries	Cupful	Raspberries, grapes
Stewed/canned fruit	Three serving spoons	Stewed apple, canned peaches
Dried fruit	Half serving spoon	Apricots, raisins
Fruit juice	Full wine glass	Orange juice, fresh
VEGETABLES		
Green vegetables	Two serving spoons	Broccoli, spinach
Root vegetables	Two serving spoons	Carrots, parsnips
Very small vegetables	Three serving spoons	Peas, sweet corn
Pulses and beans	Two serving spoons	Baked beans, kidney beans
Salad	Bowl	Lettuce, tomato

*A portion is equal to approximately 80 grams or almost 3 ounces.
From *British Medical Journal* 1995;310.

Currently there is a definite movement away from meat and toward vegetarian diets. Studies show that those eating meatless diets have much lower risks of dying from cancer or from any cause. Nutritionally sound vegetarian diets have definite benefits over diets that include animal foods. Several variations of strict vegetarian diets are both attractive and healthful.

It is important that those wishing to continue meat consumption recognize that incorporating lean cuts of red meat (beef, veal, and pork) into their diets will have some of the same lipid lowering benefits of white meat (poultry and fish) according to a recent study. This news allows for greater flexibility in and possibly improved patient acceptance of lipid-lowering diets. As a point of fact, however, white meat does have fewer calories, less total fat, and less saturated fat than the same size or weight portion of red meat or dark poultry. Cholesterol content is similar for all except fish, which is generally lower in cholesterol.

What About Other Items in the Diet?

EGGS

The authors had little, and certainly nothing good, to say about egg consumption in the first edition of this book. One reason is that one egg contains 213 mg of cholesterol, an important fact considering that the total daily recommended allowance for cholesterol is 300 mg. In recent years, however, researchers have tried to make eggs more heart-friendly by enriching them with omega-3 fatty acids or developing processes that lower cholesterol contents of eggs. Currently, these efforts have not met with much success. An egg is still a good source of inexpensive protein and nutrients, and it is not as harmful as the saturated fats found in many meats in causing high blood levels of cholesterol. Two recent and rather large studies of egg consumption came to some surprising conclusions. Except for diabetics, who still must limit their egg intakes, people who ate one egg daily were no more likely to develop heart disease than those who ate less than one egg per week. Eggs are capable of raising total and LDL cholesterol levels and should be limited for those with known high cholesterol levels, especially if they already have coronary artery disease; but for those who eat an otherwise healthy low-fat diet, an occasional egg may not be as harmful as once thought.

SODIUM

The body actually needs little sodium (less than one-fourth teaspoon) each day. It appears reasonable to avoid excess salt in the diet, especially if blood pressure levels are borderline or elevated. Salt is also a problem for the obese and those who tend to retain fluids.

CARBOHYDRATES

Up to 60 percent of total daily calories should come from carbohydrates, which are of three types: sugars, starches, and fiber. Carbohydrates provide the fuel that the body needs in order to function.

The carbohydrate portion of a healthy diet is best composed mostly of starches and especially fibers (i.e., grains, breads, pastas, cereals, potatoes, and corn) rather than sugars (e.g., candy, jelly, soda, pastries, and cookies), which can blunt the appetite for the former and contribute to the elevation of blood-fat levels.

PROTEIN

The average American eats far more protein than is needed. The body's daily protein requirement is 0.36 grams per pound of body weight, which calculates to 54 grams of protein daily for a person weighing 150 pounds. As with excess calories from carbohydrates, excess calories from protein can end up as additions to fat stores. Also, it is recognized that a high-protein diet often is a high-fat diet. Examples of common protein sources include:

1 cup milk	8 g
1 egg	7 g
1 oz. hard cheese	7 g
3 oz. meat, poultry, or fish	21 g
1 cup yogurt	8 to 11 g

SOY

Soybeans are legumes. They are rich in fiber and free of cholesterol and contain monounsaturated and polyunsaturated fats, omega-3 fatty acids, and all eight essential amino acids. Diets high in soy are associated with low cholesterol levels and beneficial effects on blood vessels when soy products are substituted for meat in the diet and because their components have estrogen-like effects and antioxidant capabilities. Soy foods are available as tofu (which is made from the liquid extracted from processed soybeans), soy milk, meat substitutes, and a tasty soy butter. It is valuable to incorporate soy products into the daily diet.

NUTS

Nuts can be valuable to a healthy diet. Though nuts contain between 14 and 20 grams of fat per ounce, the type of fat is of beneficial monounsaturated and polyunsaturated forms and is free of cholesterol. Approximately 80 percent of the calories in most nuts come from fat. Studies have shown reductions of 8 to 12 percent in LDL cholesterol levels when certain nuts (e.g., almonds and walnuts) were substituted for saturated fats in the diet. Some suggest a satiety factor associated with eating nuts. Nuts are valuable sources of vitamin E and other vitamins, minerals, and antioxidants. Because they are high in calories, nuts are best eaten dry roasted and in 1 to 3 ounce portions only a few times per week.

BUTTER/MARGARINE SUBSTITUTES

Often called "designer" margarines, two new products, Benecol" (pine tree wood pulp-based) and Take Control" (soy-based), are good tasting and very low in saturated fat, with little, if any, cholesterol. Eaten regularly in moderate amounts, these products are associated with reasonably good (10 to 15 percent) lowering of LDL cholesterol levels. They decrease intestinal absorption and increase fecal excretion of both dietary and biliary cholesterol.

OLIVE OIL

Olive oil is a valued and tasty replacement for butter and meat. Important to remember, however, is its high calorie content of 120 calories per tablespoon.

COFFEE

Coffee probably is not much of a health risk if no more than five cups per day are consumed, unless individuals have special sensitivities to caffeine products.

Diet Planning Considerations

In planning diets and preparing meals, it is important to estimate correct serving sizes. Being able to do this is especially helpful when eating in restaurants. The following associations may be of use:

Food	Approximate Serving Sizes
1 cup	Size of a woman's fist
1-½ cup	Size of a man's fist
3 oz. meat, fish, or poultry	Deck of cards
1-½ oz. cheese	Pair of dice
1 tsp. oil	Size of tip of thumb
1 cup dry cereal	Large handful
1 medium piece, fruit	Baseball
1 potato serving	Tennis ball
1 gram weight	Equal to weight of a paperclip

Recommendations

1. Follow a dietary program that allows you to maintain desirable weight.
2. Familiarize yourself with the Food Guide Pyramid.
3. Reduce meat and fat in your diet.
4. Eat at least five portions of fruits and vegetables each day.
5. Whenever possible, substitute unsaturated for saturated fat.
6. Consider adding soy products to your diet.
7. Watch out for and avoid trans-fats.

Recommendations from the American Heart Association

The American Heart Association recommends that those with elevated blood cholesterol levels follow Step I or Step II diets as advised by their physicians.

STEP I DIET

On a Step I diet, patients should eat:

- Thirty percent or less daily total calories from fat
- Eight to 10 percent daily total calories from saturated fat
- Less than 300 mg of dietary cholesterol per day
- Just enough calories to achieve and maintain healthy weight. The physician or dietitian can determine an individual's reasonable calorie level

Patients whose blood cholesterol levels are not lowered sufficiently using the Step I diet or who are at high risk for heart disease should switch to the Step II diet. Patients with heart disease should start with the Step II diet.

STEP II DIET

On a Step II diet, patients should eat:

- Thirty percent or less daily total calories from fat
- Less than seven percent daily total calories from saturated fat
- Less than 200 mg of dietary cholesterol per day
- Just enough calories to achieve and maintain a health weight. The physician or dietitian can determine an individual's reasonable calorie level

Further Reading

Williams C: Healthy eating: Clarifying advice about fruits and vegetables. Br Med J 1995;310.

Exercise:
Physical and Mental Benefits

If we could give every individual the right amount of exercise, not too little and not too much, we would have found the safest way to health.

-Hippocrates

Facts

1. About 24 percent of Americans ages 18 and older report no leisure time physical activities.

2. Among people ages 55 and older, 38 percent report essentially sedentary lifestyles.

3. It has been estimated that about 12 percent of all mortality in the U.S. is related to lack of regular physical activity.

4. Regular strenuous leisure time exercise in middle-aged men can decrease the risk of cardiac arrest by up to 65 percent and that of sudden heart attack by up to 30 percent.

5. Exercise can reduce total mortality and cardiac mortality by 20 to 25 percent in patients with coronary artery disease.

6. Routine exercise programs have proven valuable for a variety of mental and emotional problems.

7. Estimates suggest that only about 38 percent of women exercise regularly.

Each year in the U.S., as many as 250,000 deaths are attributed to lack of regular physical activity. Many studies have shown that physical activity reduces risks of many diseases such as:

- Heart disease
- High blood pressure
- Cancer
- Osteoporosis
- Diabetes mellitus
- Stroke

The exact manner in which exercise exerts its many beneficial effects is unknown, but important associations and long-term benefits of exercise have been recognized and confirmed. Exercise has been associated with lower blood pressures and improved blood fat profiles than are found for sedentary individuals. Exercise:

- Increases HDL cholesterol levels
- Lowers triglyceride levels
- Sometimes decreases LDL cholesterol levels
- Helps control weight
- Reduces blood pressure
- Helps relieve stress
- Improves the work capacity of the heart

It also appears to be able to delay onset of heart disease and, should a heart attack occur, improve survival rates. In one study, the risk of heart attack was reduced by as much as 50 percent in active compared to sedentary men.

In a London study of middle-aged conductors of double-decker buses, conductors who constantly ran from the lower to upper decks and down again had smaller waist sizes and developed much less coronary artery disease than sedentary bus drivers.

Exercise also appears to be able to reduce risks of potentially dangerous blood clots forming in the body under certain conditions and of heart irregularities by other mechanisms. It can also improve functional work capacity and help control body weight.

For many years, physical inactivity has been recognized as a contributor to development of coronary artery disease. More recently, however, a sedentary lifestyle has been noted as a major risk factor for coronary artery disease, along with other risk factors, including:

⊙ High blood pressure
⊙ Hypercholesterolemia
⊙ Cigarette smoking

Though most earlier studies were conducted using male subjects, recent studies suggest that physical activity also offers cardiovascular protection for women. One study found a 44-percent reduction in risk of heart attack associated with regular exercise in women. Recent studies have also suggested that elderly subjects who exercised developed disability at a much slower rate than those who did not, despite the fact that those who exercised had higher rates of fractures and short-term problems related to exercise behaviors. Those in the exercise group also had lower mortality.

The benefits of exercise are not limited to the heart. Patients with peripheral vascular disease can significantly improve their walking ability by engaging in exercise programs. Studies show that exercise protects against:

○ Colon cancer
○ Development of noninsulin-dependent diabetes
○ Osteoporosis
○ Mental health disorders
○ Breast cancer
○ Symptomatic gallstone disease in men

Exercise not only is important in preventing but also is useful in treating osteoporosis, along with other therapies. Weight-bearing activities such as walking, jogging, and climbing stairs and weight-lifting and back-strengthening exercises all have value.

The problem of lack of exercise is particularly important in the U.S., where it includes 20 to 30 percent of the population. This statistic indicates that 35 to 50 million Americans are at a two- to fourfold increased risk for cardiovascular mortality. Only about 22 percent of American adults meet or exceed recently recommended exercise guidelines. About 54 percent are involved in some physical activity but not enough to meet guidelines; 24 percent are sedentary and do little if any exercise. In the latter group, it has been estimated that as much as 35 percent of excess coronary artery disease could be eliminated if these people became more physically active.

The question is, how much exercise is enough? Current recommendations from the Centers for Disease Control and Prevention and the American College of Sports Medicine are that every adult in the U.S. accumulate about 30 minutes of moderately intense physical activity preferably every day. This can be accomplished in one effort or from several shorter bouts of activity during the course of a day. A brisk walk (at a rate of three to four miles per hour) is a good standard. Walking has an added advantage (over swimming or cycling, for example) in that it is a weight-bearing exercise and, thus, is able to increase bone density, mostly in the legs and spine. Other activities, e.g., dancing, climbing stairs, and cycling, can be substituted according to personal desires and preferences. The goal is to expend at least 200 extra calories each day by exercising.

Some studies show that significant health benefits are achievable at exercise levels that exceed current minimum guidelines (e.g., running up to 50 miles per week), though certain risks and a variety of injuries can also occur with such vigorous programs. Because of proven benefits of a moderate amount of physical activity, experts recommend that most adults pursue moderate-intensity exercise programs.

Recent studies also suggest hope for those who cannot fit a structured exercise program into their lives. In these studies, individuals were able to accumulate adequate periods of moderate-intensity activity during the day by, for example, taking longer walks on the way to office meetings, walking around airports while waiting for flights, walking around soccer fields at their children's games, and parking the car farther from the office.

Studies showing a reduced incidence of breast cancer related to exercise appear to require four or more hours a week of vigorous exercise (e.g., involvements in competitive sports) for that benefit to occur. Moderate exercise (e.g., walking or bicycling for similar periods of time) was not associated with reduction in risk for breast cancer.

Lifting weights is also valuable, even for individuals in their 90s. Weight-training programs can improve strength and balance in these individuals, increase muscle mass, and even result in improved walking capabilities. Benefits accrue from weight-lifting sessions of at least two days per week, with such sessions consisting of 10 to 15 repetitions of 10 sets of various exercises.

Many commercially available books and pamphlets can provide specific amounts and/or durations of favorite activities required for specific benefits (e.g., 20 minutes of jogging burns about 200 calories). Current exercise recommendations are considered minimum suggestions.

It appears that, within reason, the more exercise performed, the better and the lower the risks of disabilities and death from coronary artery disease. One study suggested that men in the 60 to 80 age group who walked approximately two miles per day lived five years longer than those who walked less than one mile per day. The large Harvard Alumni Health Study has shown that, at any given quantity of energy expenditure, death rates were significantly lower with moderately vigorous rather than less vigorous physical activities.

A recent report from Stanford University suggests that older persons ages 50 to 72 who engage in vigorous running and other aerobic activities have lower mortality rates and slower development of disabilities than members of the general population. Exercise and strength-training sessions have been shown to be beneficial even for those ages 75 and older. It is hoped that such activities for this

population will result in:
- Improved:
  - Ambulation
  - Balance
  - Coordination
- Fewer falls
- Better abilities to maintain independent lifestyles

Exercise is important for maintaining good balance, walking being one of the best exercises for achieving that goal. As individuals age and become less active, they lose muscle strength in the legs, which is needed for maintaining balancing skills.

Some have expressed concerns about possible development of cardiac problems during vigorous exercise; however, about 96 percent of heart attacks occur during rest, with only four percent related to vigorous exertion. Also, of those who have heart attacks during vigorous exertion, the majority had been sedentary or were among those who exercised infrequently. Those who exercised regularly had an overall lower risk of heart attack.

Recommendations
1. Walk briskly for at least one-half hour six to seven days per week.
2. Continue an exercise program throughout your life.
3. If you have medical problems, disabilities, or other limitations, seek a physician's advice and guidance in initiating and developing any exercise program.
4. If you are able, choose a more vigorous physical activity program for added benefits.

5. Even if you are unable to increase activities to desired or recommended levels, any increase is beneficial and can reduce risks of coronary artery disease.
6. Seek activities you enjoy; you are more likely to stick with them.

Further Reading

Fries JF, Singh G, et al.: Running and the development of disability with age. Ann Int Med October 1994.

Sleep:
Importance to Personal Health

Sleeping is no mean art. For its sake, one must stay awake all day.

-Neitzsche

Facts

1. Up to five percent of middle-aged men have sleep apnea.

2. Automobile accidents occur about two to three times more often in individuals with sleep apnea.

3. The incidence of heart attack is about five times greater in patients who snore and have sleep apnea.

4. Individuals with sleep apnea are at about three times greater risk of stroke.

5. Studies have shown that cigarette smokers are significantly more likely than nonsmokers to report problems going to sleep and staying asleep and daytime sleepiness.

6. Fifty-five percent of vehicle accidents in which drivers fell asleep involve people younger than age 25.

Sleep occupies a significant portion of the average day. At some time or other, most people have complaints of difficulty falling asleep and staying asleep or not feeling rested after sleep. Some people feel excessively sleepy during the day without realizing that something might be wrong with their sleep.

Transient problems with sleep, often associated with various identifiable factors, are recognized and usually managed by individuals. Chronic problems, however, often are undiagnosed and, thus, left untreated; because their importance is unrecognized, these problems do not get reported to physicians.

It is a common thing for individuals to fall asleep while driving and become involved in traffic accidents. Probably most of these victims are healthy people who are sleep-deprived due to lifestyle or work schedules, though many may have long-standing sleep disorders (e.g., sleep apnea) that interfere with sleep on a regular basis and cause subsequent loss of daytime alertness and increased risks of automobile accidents. Also, some individuals may take medications that have sedating effects or that disrupt routine sleeping patterns.

Patients must discuss sleep problems with their physicians. Sleep complaints suggest several important causes, including:

- Psychiatric illnesses (often depression)
- Major medical illnesses, especially those involving the:
  - Thyroid gland
  - Heart
  - Lung

○ Illnesses associated with pain, as well as problems related to the medicines used for its treatment

A large variety of nonprescription and prescription drugs can interfere with sleep; these include:

○ Nonprescription (over-the-counter):
  ○ Pseudoephedrine
  ○ Phenylpropanolamine
  ○ Diphenhydramine
  ○ Chlorpheniramine
  ○ Caffeine in drugs (e.g., Anacin®, Excedrin® and Empirin®)
○ Prescription:
  ○ Antidepressants (amitriptyline, doxepin)
  ○ Propranolol
  ○ Metoprolol
  ○ Clonidine
  ○ Bronchodilators (inhalers)
  ○ Phenytoin
  ○ Progesterone
  ○ Corticosteroids
  ○ Methyldopa
  ○ Nonsteroidal anti-inflammatory agents

This side effect may occur only in some individuals or under certain circumstances and, thus, may not have been anticipated. Alcohol, caffeine, and even some medications thought to help sleep can cause sleep problems for certain individuals. Caffeine can be a particular problem for some who are especially sensitive to its effects, which can remain in the body for up to 20 hours. For such people, even a single cup of coffee in the morning could prove to be problematic. Some individuals may have to avoid caffeine completely, even that found in tea, colas, and chocolate.

Sleep problems are even more common in the elderly and become more prominent with advancing age. Older individuals with sleep problems can be bothered during the day with:

- ○ Fatigue
- ○ Impaired thinking
- ○ Decline in motor skill capabilities
- ○ Decreased alertness

These effects are problematic when this or any population drives or works with potentially dangerous machinery. Reasonable estimates suggest that about 15 to 20 percent of all motor vehicle accidents are attributable to sleepiness. In the U.S., this would account for up to 7,000 fatalities each year.

Fatigue also has been recognized as the leading cause of trucking crashes. Impairment in performance caused by sleep deprivation has been compared to impairment caused by alcohol. Sustained wakefulness for 17 hours can decrease performance similar to drinking as much as two (1½ oz.) drinks of alcohol.

Good medications, when used appropriately and under a physician's care, can be helpful in treating insomnia. One must be concerned with the half-life of such medications (i.e., the time it takes for the medicine to be cleared from the body); shorter half-life drugs are less likely to have carry-over sedation that affects daytime functioning. Also, toxicity of the drug is important because of the higher risks of overdosing with some preparations. Commonly used and effective drugs include:

- Estazolam (ProSom®)
- Flurazepam (Dalmane®)
- Quazepam (Doral®)
- Temazepam (Restoril®)
- Triazolam (Halcion®)
- Zaleplon (Sonata®)
- Zolpidem (Ambien®)

Such drugs should be used only for short periods because of risks of developing dependency and withdrawal symptoms when discontinuing their use. They should not be used for chronic insomnia because of their potential addictive qualities and because they can mask underlying medical problems. Alcohol should not be consumed when sleeping agents are being taken, and these agents should be avoided if sleep apnea is suspected.

Some individuals find use of nonprescription sleep aids helpful. Available aids include:
- Diphenhydramine:
  - Nytol®
  - Sleep-Eze®
  - Sominex®
  - Tylenol PM®
  - Anacin PM®
  - Excedrin PM®
- Doxylamine:
  - Unisom®

These products contain a sedating antihistamine and, as with use of prescription drugs, must be used with care. Even if taken at night, they can cause daytime drowsiness, which can make driving and other tasks risky. Melatonin, though commonly touted as a sleep aid, does not have sufficient data to support its use in that role; there also is not enough data about melatonin's potential complications and toxicity.

The most serious sleeping disorder is sleep apnea, a relatively common disorder seen in about two percent of women and four percent of men (about two to five million people in the U.S.). In sleep apnea, individuals stop breathing up to hundreds of times each night during sleep. An excess of 10 such events per hour are generally necessary to establish diagnosis. These individuals are often unaware of their apnea and often do not suspect any sleep problem.

Sleep apnea tends to be more common in the elderly; to some degree, it occurs in 25 percent of people ages 60 and older. It also is associated with obesity and high blood pressure. Certain airway obstruction problems may be found in such individuals.

Symptoms of sleep apnea include:
- Snoring
- Daytime sleepiness
- Early morning headache
- Memory changes
- Thought deficits
- Depression

These symptoms often are overlooked, though loud snoring, choking noises, and disruptions of breathing noted by sleeping partners may be the best clue to sleep apnea.

As occurs with other sleep disorders, sleep apnea patients have a higher frequency of automobile accidents. More important problems, however, result from poor oxygenation of the blood during periods

of disrupted breathing, including:
- Heart attack
- Stroke
- Sudden death

Complicating the ability to diagnose sleep apnea is the fact that symptoms often are misinterpreted as anxiety or depression or the results of aging. Additionally, many physicians are unfamiliar with the disorder and the varied and confusing forms that it can manifest.

There are specific, effective, and often lifesaving treatments for sleep apnea and the diseases that may be associated with it.

Recommendations

1. Recognize that sleep disorders exist and can have serious consequences.
2. Recognize that lifestyle factors (e.g., smoking, alcohol, and drugs) can interfere with sleep.
3. Seek your partner's observations of your nighttime snoring or breathing habits.
4. Be suspicious of any medications you take as possible causes of or contributors to sleeping disorders.
5. If you are suspicious of sleep apnea, avoid sleeping on your back; elevating the head of the bed may also help.
6. Any suspicion of a sleep disorder should be brought to the attention of a physician who is knowledgeable about and interested in the condition.
7. Lack of response to therapies, suspicion of repeated sleep disorder-related accidents, or a picture suggesting sleep apnea or its complications should trigger a request for an evaluation at a recognized sleep disorder center.

Vitamins and Supplements: Which Are Necessary for Health Maintenance and Which Are Unnecessary and Even Dangerous?

Life loves to be taken by the lapels and told, "I am with you, kid. Let's go."

-Maya Angelou

Facts

1. Many Americans take vitamin supplements, though most do not need them.

2. Vitamins taken in excess of the Recommended Daily Allowances can be harmful.

3. Mineral requirements can easily be met with a balanced, varied diet.

4. Studies do not show that healthy persons who take nutrient supplements experience increased energy or added disease protection.

5. The American Dietetic Association advocates that food is the best source of nutrients and that eating well-balanced diets provides a unique balance of nutrients that cannot be duplicated by any combinations of vitamin and mineral supplements.

6. Antioxidants, including vitamin E, are probably without enough scientific support for their routine use. They do not decrease cardiac mortality and could possibly prove harmful, as has occurred with use of beta-carotene in certain settings.

Millions of Americans take vitamin and mineral supplements, responding to suggestions by supplement manufacturers that their products can prolong life, increase energy, prevent cancers and heart disease, improve sexual prowess, and ward off disease.

Guidelines for vitamin requirements are set by the Food and Nutrition Board of the National Research Council and termed Recommended Dietary Allowances (RDAs). These recommendations exceed the needs of most healthy people, but avoid the excesses that can be potentially harmful.

Most adults in this country should not require vitamin and mineral supplements because their diets probably provide adequate nutrient intake. Essential nutrients can be obtained from balanced and varied diets that contain:

- Lots of fruits and vegetables
- Grains
- Some dairy products
- Lean meat
- Skinless poultry
- Fish

Obtaining necessary nutrients from the diet avoids problems related to excess vitamin and mineral intake yet provides the various known and unknown materials in foods that assist and/or enhance the actions of vitamins, minerals, and other materials found in foods.

Significant problems can result from excessive doses of:
- Vitamin A
- Vitamin C
- Vitamin E
- Folate
- Vitamin B_6
- Niacin
- Selenium
- Zinc
- Calcium
- Iron

Some people do require daily multiple vitamin and/or mineral supplements. For those who need them, the supplements are safe if they contain no more than 150 percent of RDAs for each component. Individuals most likely to benefit from supplements include:
- Dieters consuming fewer than 1,200 calories daily
- Individuals with malabsorption syndromes
- Elderly people who:
  - Appear malnourished
  - Have poor diets
  - Have poor appetites
- Individuals with specific vitamin or mineral deficiencies as suggested by a manifest disease process
- Alcoholics
- Smokers
- Pregnant and nursing women
- Individuals taking drugs that distort the appetite
- Strict vegetarians
- Individuals with kidney failure, especially if on dialysis
- Elderly people with poor sunlight exposure

○ Most postmenopausal women, who need calcium supplements

○ Menstruating women, who may need iron supplements

○ Individuals taking orlistat (Xenical®) for weight reduction

All vitamin supplements, with the exception of Vitamin B_{12}, are chemically produced by a manufacturing process that yields both the desired natural form of the vitamin supplement as well as undesirable chemical products, which, in high doses, can be harmful. Thus, the safety factor achieved by acquiring the true natural forms of vitamin supplements as they are found in foods becomes apparent.

Unfortunately, diets of many elderly Americans may not provide desirable amounts of certain beneficial vitamins; thus, inexpensive, multivitamin tablets are seen as valuable for this population. Often the best buy is from a reputable, generic manufacturer, but consumers must be certain that the USP designation is on the label and that it is best that multivitamin preparations be taken with a meal.

Although age-related changes in elderly persons can bring about this potential need for vitamin supplements, fortified food products can also provide specific needed vitamins. Useful daily supplements and dosages for elderly consumers should contain:

○ Folic acid – 400 ug

○ Vitamin B_{12} - 2.4 ug

○ Vitamin B_6 - 1.5 to 1.7 mg

○ Riboflavin - 1.1 to 1.3 mg

○ Vitamin D – 400 to 600 IU

A fair percentage of older Americans have atrophic gastritis with low acid production, making it difficult for these people to obtain and absorb vitamin B_{12} and, thus, contributing to deficiency problems. Additionally, this population's aging skin is less efficient in converting UV light to vitamin D, which also contributes to deficiency. Elderly individuals, who often do not drink enough milk and are not exposed to sunlight, will likely need vitamin D supplements.

Vitamin C and certainly beta-carotene supplements are probably not needed by individuals who eat reasonable diets. The average American diet, for example, offers about 17 IU of vitamin E, while the RDA is 30 IU. Doses ranging from 100 to 800 IU daily are used in efforts to lower risks of heart disease. Though these doses are safe for most individuals, they can present serious problems for those taking blood thinners. The American Heart Association does not endorse vitamin E supplements and cannot conclude that vitamin E reduces risks or mortality rates of coronary artery disease. More studies are needed before recommendations can be made.

Much interest has been generated by the possibility that beta-carotene and vitamins C and E may help prevent cancer and heart disease because of their antioxidant qualities. At present, however, the best recommendation is that more of the natural foods that contain these antioxidants (e.g., fruits, vegetables, and grains) be included in the diet. The American Heart Association does not yet find enough evidence to recommend antioxidant supplementation for the general public.

Adequate blood concentrations of antioxidant vitamins that are associated with improved health status can be acquired by appropriate dietary intake, but high doses of antioxidants can be associated with significant health problems. One study of vitamin E supplementation showed an unexpected increase in risks of death from hemorrhagic stroke. Another study of beta-carotene supplementation showed an unexpected increase in mortality from lung cancer and coronary artery disease. In many studies in which increased antioxidant intake was shown to be correlated with reduced disease risks, the intake was from antioxidant-rich foods rather than vitamin supplementation.

There has been some recent interest in lycopene, a phytochemical with potent antioxidant properties that is found in tomatoes, especially cooked tomatoes. Lycopene-rich foods appear to reduce risks of heart attack and prostate cancer; this phenomenon certainly deserves watching for confirmatory results.

The authors often see patients who take pills or powdered preparations that are "concentrates" of fruits and vegetables. These are marketed aggressively to patients who wish to be certain they receive all important nutrients in their diets. Such products, however, often do not provide valuable fiber or some nutrients that are readily found in the food items they represent. The convenience of these products is hardly worth their lesser values and often great costs.

Despite numerous and varied claims for mineral supplements, healthy people who eat appropriate numbers of calories in varied diets that include plenty of fruits, vegetables, and grains can easily achieve the recommended intake of minerals, which include:

- Calcium
- Selenium
- Iron
- Zinc
- Chromium
- Iodine
- Phosphorus
- Cobalt
- Copper
- Fluoride
- Manganese
- Molybdenum

Taken in excess, individual minerals or combinations of them can cause problems, including toxicity. Toxicity is not expected from eating natural foods that contain these minerals.

The exception to this rule is calcium. To protect against osteoporosis, increased incidences of fractures in the elderly, and associated increased mortality, calcium supplements may be required. The elderly, due to dietary deficiencies and/or a lack of sunlight exposure, may be deficient in calcium and vitamin D. (See Chapter 6 for recommended dosages of calcium supplements.) Dairy products (e.g., skim milk [300 mg calcium per cup]) are the best sources of dietary calcium. For those unable to ingest enough dietary calcium, supplements (e.g., calcium carbonate or calcium citrate taken two or three times daily with meals) are beneficial. Daily vitamin D recommendations for men and women are:

- Ages 19 to 50 - 200 IU
- Ages 51 to 70 – 400 IU
- Ages 71 and older – 600 IU

Even higher doses may be beneficial in the elderly who are ill or are taking steroids. Vitamin D supplementation, along with calcium, in the elderly has the potential to reduce rates of hip and other fractures and also helps prevent osteoporosis, partly because it stimulates calcium absorption from the intestine.

It is amazing what individuals are willing to ingest in efforts to achieve healthier and longer lives, avoid problems associated with natural aging, and restore qualities and feelings associated with youth. Manufacturers of supplements, health foods, and natural products claim benefits for which there are no supporting evidence, no FDA approvals, and usually no scientific bases. Often these items are expensive and by themselves can be dangerous or prove to be especially toxic when combined with other drugs or products. Additionally, there is inadequate knowledge about problems associated with long-term ingestion of these items.

Recommendations

1. Obtain vitamins and minerals by eating a balanced diet that includes at least five servings of fruits, vegetables, and grains daily.
2. A simple, inexpensive multiple vitamin/mineral supplement based on RDAs may benefit certain groups (see above).
3. Avoid vitamin/mineral supplements in dosages greater than RDA recommendations.
4. You may need calcium supplements, depending on your age, gender, and dietary calcium intake.
5. A reasonable and effective way to obtain necessary antioxidants is to eat a variety of fruits and vegetables of different colors (green, orange, red, and yellow).

Further Reading

Barrett S, Herbert V: *The Vitamin Pushers.* Prometheus Books, 1994.

Aspirin:
The Magic Potion?

The desire to take medicine is perhaps the greatest feature which distinguishes man from animals.

-William Osler

Facts

1. For those who have had heart attacks, aspirin could reduce risks of having another by 30 percent.

2. It appears that people who take aspirin are less likely to die from cancers of the colon, rectum, stomach, and esophagus.

3. If you feel you are having a heart attack, chew an aspirin tablet while calling for medical help.

Aspirin is an important drug with many uses. Potential beneficial effects of aspirin intake in people with heart disease, stroke, and certain blood vessel problems and people who might develop certain cancers suggest a role for this drug in life extension.

Though aspirin has many potential beneficial effects, its widespread usage is limited by a variety of significant side effects that include:

- Peptic ulcers
- Gastritis
- Hemorrhages in the:
  - Upper gastrointestinal tract
  - Urinary tract
  - Bowel
  - Brain
- Allergic reactions (occasionally)

Even low doses of aspirin (81 mg) can cause gastric discomfort and, though rare, gastrointestinal or brain hemorrhage. Though the desired effects of aspirin are seen across a wide range of doses, side effects increase with higher doses. Aspirin is a common cause of skin bruising, though this effect is no reason to terminate use. A recent study suggests that there is no significant difference in the rates of upper gastrointestinal bleeding with use of regular or more expensive enteric-coated or buffered aspirin forms.

Aspirin can also be a problem for those with uncontrolled hypertension and for alcoholics because of hemorrhagic stroke and gastrointestinal bleeding, respectively.

Aspirin is effective for those with coronary artery disease and those who have had or are at increased risks for heart attack. It is especially useful in lowering risks of death (by 50 percent) and heart attack in patients in the process of having heart attacks. The American Heart Association estimates that 5,000 to 10,000 lives could be saved each year if those experiencing chest pain or other symptoms of heart attack take an aspirin (preferably chewed at the first sign of symptoms). The aspirin prevents blood clots from forming in the coronary artery by making blood platelets less sticky. It also is known to have numerous nonplatelet-related effects, and its anti-inflammatory ability appears to be a factor in the treatment and prevention of coronary artery disease.

Following a heart attack or medical condition that enhances risks for heart attack or stroke, a daily aspirin (325 mg) or even a baby aspirin (81 mg) is of proven benefit. Taking aspirin after a heart attack lowers rates of death and recurrent heart attack by 20 percent. Patients with angina pectoris or coronary bypass grafts also benefit from taking aspirin.

Use of aspirin in middle-aged or older men who, because of risk factors, are at great risk for a first heart attack may be beneficial, but potential side effects may negate the desired value. In fact, in men without symptoms or risk factors for coronary artery disease, aspirin may prove more harmful than beneficial. Because of its potential adverse effects, aspirin is not approved for decreasing heart attack risks in healthy individuals. If it is used, probably low-dose (one baby aspirin) each day taken with food will provide benefit while minimizing risks.

Studies have shown a benefit of aspirin in reducing risks of stroke in patients with symptoms (e.g., transient ischemic attacks [TIAs]) but not much benefit in asymptomatic individuals. Aspirin may have some benefit in reducing stroke that is associated with certain heart rhythm disorders (e.g., atrial fibrillation).

Aspirin appears to have some anticancer effects in the digestive tract, especially the large bowel, when taken for many years. The data are still not strong enough, however, in view of potential aspirin complications, for recommendations of routine use for this purpose to be made.

Recommendations

1. Take aspirin (dose as recommended by your physician) if you have coronary artery disease and especially if you have poorly controlled symptoms of it or have had a heart attack.
2. Take aspirin (under a physician's guidance) if you have symptoms or signs suggesting an impending stroke (TIA) or after a completed stroke.
3. Avoid aspirin if you are already taking other blood thinners, have or are prone to peptic ulcers, or have other potential bleeding problems.
4. Use the lowest dose of aspirin that is known to be effective for the condition under treatment.

Estrogen and Progesterone: Benefits and Dangers

There is a fountain of youth: it is your mind, your talents, the creativity you bring to your life and the lives of people you love. When you learn to tap this resource, you will truly have defeated old age.

-Sophia Loren

Facts

1. In the U.S., a postmenopausal woman is 10 times more likely to die from coronary artery disease than from breast cancer.

2. Estrogen replacement therapy could reduce the risk of hip fracture in women by as much as 25 to 50 percent.

3. Studies suggest that smoking has an antiestrogen effect.

4. Studies suggest that estrogen may delay onset and decrease risks of Alzheimer's disease in postmenopausal women.

5. Estrogen is the most effective agent for the prevention of postmenopausal osteoporosis.

With vast numbers of women at or approaching menopause, it is important that interventions that might reduce or prevent long-term effects of estrogen deficiency, namely coronary artery disease and osteoporosis, be considered. After menopause, blood fat patterns change significantly, with increases in LDL and decreases in HDL cholesterol levels. These and other changes can eventually result in the development of coronary artery disease that will occur in about one-half of women, with about 30 percent dying from heart disease.

Estrogen/progesterone hormone therapy appears to be the answer, although not all studies agree on this point and more data are needed. Women taking hormones are at some modest increased risk for developing blood clots and gallbladder disease. However, estrogen does have recognized cardioprotective effects that do not appear to be negated by the addition of progesterone to the regimen, which lowers the increased risk of endometrial cancer associated with estrogen use alone. At present, it is thought that the best approach is to recommend that women with coronary artery disease not initiate hormone replacement therapy, though those already on such treatments should not discontinue it but be monitored closely.

For women without coronary artery disease, hormone replacement therapy should be considered not only for its cardioprotective benefits but also for its benefits associated with severe menopausal symptoms, osteoporosis prevention, and other potential noncoronary benefits. Personal or strong family histories of breast cancer and/or venous thromboembolism are important factors to be considered for all women considering initiating hormone therapy. Until the many questions about hormone replacement are answered, women should take conventional steps to help reduce the heart disease risks that occur after menopause.

A relatively new drug, raloxifene (Evista®), targets estrogen receptors in certain tissues (e.g., bone) and has been used to prevent osteoporosis and vertebral fractures. The drug was originally developed as a potential treatment for breast cancer and has shown no evidence of increased breast or endometrial cancer risks. It does show some of the lipid profile-improving qualities of hormone replacement therapy, but its cardioprotective effects are still under study. Though appearing to have a low side effect profile, it cannot be used to treat hot flashes and may, in fact, precipitate them. The drug also appears to be similar to estrogen in increasing risks of blood clots. It appears to be establishing its role in treating certain groups of women at risk for osteoporosis.

Declining estrogen levels in postmenopausal women results in hundreds of thousands of osteoporosis-related fractures. These hip and spine fractures, which can be crippling, occur in about one-half of all postmenopausal women who live into their 80s. Estrogen replacement therapy could reduce risks of hip fracture in women by as much as 25 to 50 percent. Women most likely to benefit from estrogen are those:

○ With early or surgical menopause
○ With multiple cardiac risk factors, especially blood fat abnormalities

○ At increased risks for osteoporosis or fractures, such as those who:
  ○ Smoke
  ○ Have family histories of fractures
  ○ Are thin
  ○ Have been on lengthy courses of cortisone preparations

Some women should not have estrogen therapy. This group includes women with prior breast cancer and/or histories of estrogen-related complications (e.g., blood clots) or liver disease.

There are some side effects of estrogen therapy. These include endometrial cancer, if estrogen is given without progesterone, and a possible increased risk of breast cancer. However, in spite of large numbers of women being treated with estrogen replacement therapy for many years, there still is a lack of strong, convincing evidence of the association between estrogen and breast cancer risks. Counseling and close follow-up by physicians is necessary for the duration of any estrogen treatment program, especially for women who have not had hysterectomies.

For women who have had hysterectomies, estrogen is best used alone. Uterine cancer occurs in about 2.6 percent of white women ages 50 and older. Estrogen use in postmenopausal women significantly increases risks of uterine cancer and that risk increases with dose and duration of treatment.

Progesterone, often given with estrogen in women who still have uteri, eliminates excess risk of uterine cancer. The *possible small increase* in risk of breast cancer with estrogen alone may be significantly increased by the addition of progesterone according to some recent reports. More information, and consideration of a variety of treatment programs for progesterone, is needed. Your physician can help you evaluate the potential benefits and/or risks related to these therapies, and the manner and time frame in which they are used.

Progesterone is commonly associated with what are often considered to be transient side effects, such as:

○ Headache
○ Bloating
○ Irritability
○ Depression
○ Vaginal bleeding and related problems

There was also concern that the addition of progesterone might blunt the cardioprotective effects of estrogen therapy. Recent reports, however, suggest that adding progesterone to estrogen therapy does not appear to do so in relatively young postmenopausal women.

Estrogen replacement therapy in postmenopausal women may also have some value in protecting from Alzheimer's disease, colorectal cancer, and even tooth loss; but further studies are needed in these areas.

Phytoestrogens, a group of compounds found in a wide variety of plant-derived foods and drinks, have estrogenic effects, though these are weaker than natural estrogens. These compounds are under intense study and may prove to have clinical value. Unfortunately, these compounds are readily available and are commonly used in spite of inadequate knowledge of proper doses, adverse side effects, and potential toxicity. Soybean phytoestrogen has been associated with favorable effects on lipids and atherosclerosis in animals, but studies confirming its value in women are not yet available.

Recommendations

1. At the time of menopause, ask your physician about particular benefits and risks from estrogen replacement therapy for you.
2. If you are not a good candidate for estrogen replacement therapy, learn about and institute alternative regimens for avoiding osteoporosis and for reducing your risks of coronary artery disease.
3. Raloxifene (Evista®) appears to be a valuable addition to the therapeutic possibilities for postmenopausal women, particularly in preventing osteoporosis.
4. Wait for more data before embracing plant-derived estrogens.

The Physician:
How To Select Your Doctor

A physician can sometimes parry the scythe of death but has no power over the sand in the hour-glass.

-Hester Lynch Piozzi

Fact

1. A quality physician could prove to be one of the most important variables influencing life extension.

2. The physician and the patient must be a team in helping the patient live a longer and healthier life.

3. The physician is the "coach" and the patient is the "player" in the game of enhancing the quality and length of a happy life.

There is little doubt that good physicians involved in good physician/patient relationships can influence the extension of life and that the quality of that extended life should also be improved.

Much care should go into selection of personal physicians. People want physicians with whom they can feel compatible in relationships that will last for many years. Personal physicians usually are internists or family physicians. Patients must take time to find physicians they like and trust and with whom they have good personality matches.

Sometimes recommendations from friends and relatives, or especially other physicians, can put patients in contact with doctors who can be considered for the important task of overseeing health. Patients should seek physicians who, from the beginning, seem interested in them, their problems, and health maintenance. Physicians should be willing to spend a reasonable amount of time with patients during visits; after visits, patients should feel that their problems have been heard.

Obviously, patients should expect to be cared for by quality physicians with excellent reputations. Patients should feel free to check credentials of candidates.

Some may desire doctors who are listed in *Best Doctors in America* or similar publications. These physicians are often found at major university medical centers, but they often have restricted practices because of teaching and research commitments. In recent years, however, many of these doctors are spending a large percentage of their time in clinical patient care.

In seeking the right physicians, patients might consider their own special needs and specialty-related interests and skills of physician candidates. For example, internists with subspecialty interests in endocrinology might be the best match for diabetic patients. Primary physicians, however, can always direct patients to capable specialists needed to manage special problems.

Patients should note whether their personal physicians stay current with medical practices and research. This discovery will only occur with time, however, as patients determine whether they are receiving the benefits of the latest technological advances, treatments, and medicines and whether their physicians can answer questions about current media reports. It should be recognized, however, that the media often overwhelm the public with frequent reports of unimportant but interest-generating medical findings or studies. Good physicians, however, will seek pertinent information and put it into proper perspective regarding their patients' illnesses and needs.

There are numerous ways in which a physician's care can improve the quality and length of life. Good physicians will:

- Oversee patients' immunization programs, thus preventing sometimes serious or life-shortening illnesses
- Ensure proper screening studies and examinations to discover diseases at early stages when they are easier to treat
- Upon hearing patients' symptoms, quickly pursue problems and institute therapies early and effectively
- Avoid unnecessary and/or dangerous testing or procedures

- Use tried and tested medicines and treatments, always cognizant of side effects and complications
- Be concerned about potential adverse events related to combinations of drugs used in treating patients' problems
- Choose the best available consulting, surgical, or other procedure-performing specialists in an effort to achieve the best results for their patients
- Help their patients select the best hospitals, care centers, or emergency units if needed
- Guide their patients to the most effective therapy centers, rehabilitation units, and dietary and lifestyle modification programs
- Confront their patients regularly about issues such as smoking, diet, alcohol, safe sex, exercise, and cardiovascular risk factors
- Be interested in cost factors associated with evaluation and treatment, recognizing that cost-effectiveness considerations must be part of their patients' care
- Be interested in their patients' total spectrum of problems, such as anxiety, depression, or dementia, since these can trigger, mimic, cause, or exacerbate numerous other problems and result in unwanted or unexpected outcomes (e.g., suicide, accidents)
- Be advocates working in their patients' behalf when conflicts arise with health management organizations (HMOs) or other managed-care entities
- Guarantee that their practice coverage for nights, weekends, vacations, etc. is by qualified individuals who are able to meet patients' healthcare needs

It is important that there be a cooperative, understanding physician/patient relationship in order that patients might derive the greatest benefit from the association. Patients sometimes desire frequencies of visits/examinations, tests or procedures, medications, or therapies that physicians may feel are inappropriate, cost-ineffective, or potentially harmful. Today especially, physicians try to keep people out of expensive hospital settings when reasonable alternatives are available, but physicians should be willing to discuss with their patients the particular care options.

The aging of a physician's practice leads to even further demands upon his role as a health team leader and organizer. Patients may eventually need some form of supportive or custodial home care, assisted living program, nursing home care, rehabilitation program, or hospice care. Physicians, by themselves or through team efforts, should be able to direct patients toward the best programs for them and incorporate these programs into their future care situations and family, friends, and community support activities.

In recent years, more studies have begun to research interrelations between spirituality and health, and physicians are recognizing the importance of meeting the spiritual needs of their patients. As a result, physicians are beginning to understand the value of incorporating patients' spiritual and/or religious beliefs into care areas, e.g., social history portions of comprehensive patient examinations.

Recommendations

1. Use the information suggested in this chapter and take the time and effort to find the best physician match for your particular needs.

The Patient: Personal Responsibility for Wellness

The patient must combat the disease with the physician.

-Hippocrates

Facts

1. One-third of women who are prescribed estrogen replacement therapy never fill their prescriptions.

2. Of women who start estrogen replacement therapy, about one-half discontinue it within six months.

3. Forty-three percent of patients do not take long-term medications as prescribed.

4. Thirty-eight percent of patients fail to follow short-term treatment plans (e.g., taking antibiotics).

5. Up to 21 percent of prescriptions given to patients are never filled.

6. Seventy-five percent of patients do not follow lifestyle recommendations (e.g., diet and exercise programs).

7. Fifty percent of patients in post-heart attack rehabilitation programs abandon them within a year.

8. Only 30 percent of patients follow dietary recommendations after one year.

9. Of patients taking digitalis for heart failure, only 10 percent have their prescriptions filled often enough to be receiving the proper dose.

10. About half of all patients leave the doctor's office not knowing what they have been advised to do.

11. One study found that patients with heart disease who took less than 80 percent of their prescribed medications (beta-blockers) had four times the number of cardiac events (heart attack and stroke) as those who were fully adherent.

12. Up to 20 percent of patients do not present their prescriptions to a pharmacy within one month of issue.

Many of the facts presented here were noted in the September 1994 Johns Hopkins *Medical Letter* and explain why many physicians feel frustrated with problems of patient compliance. Adult patients are not compliant for a variety of reasons, discontinuing medications on their own because of:

○ Real or suspected side effects
○ Drug costs
○ Uncertainty of effectiveness
○ Vacations
○ Confusion about dose or time of dose
○ Just plain forgetfulness

Doctors, at times, contribute to the problem by:

○ Not giving patients clear instructions for taking medications
○ Not warning patients about significant or bothersome side effects
○ Making dose or time schedules too complicated
○ Not recognizing medication cost factors
○ Failing to instruct patients as to the purpose and importance of medications
○ Not dosing medications based on age, gender, kidney and liver function, other medications, and diseases to be treated

Physicians may at times fail to recognize a drug's side effect that becomes manifest when added to other drugs on a patient's program. Patients, on the other hand, take supplements, nonprescription drugs, herbs, and various other pills with unknown components in varied forms and dosages without telling their physicians. Some of these drugs can be harmful in and of themselves, in combination with other medications patients take on their own (e.g., aspirin or sinus medications), or when used alongside prescribed medications. Unfortunately, computer systems used in pharmacies are not capable of screening for potential drug interactions with herbal products.

It is becoming apparent that patients must become assertive regarding their medical care. Patients who are passive, unquestioning, and seemingly unconcerned about their medical problems are at a disadvantage, possibly receive less time and attention from their physicians and the clinic staff, and miscommunicate with their physicians by giving the impression that their condition is not as serious as it actually is. Patients should learn as much about their illnesses as possible. Resources such as books and pamphlets, especially those recommended by physicians, and the Internet all have potential value for patients to learn much about their medications, how they work, how they should be used, their side effects, and their potential complications. Patients who become more involved in their care tend to feel more confident, are less anxious about their illnesses, and are more likely to comply with and continue treatment regimens, especially regimens that are complex or uncomfortable.

Most physicians generally understand that patients, especially older patients, have spiritual needs that must be met. Studies have shown that certain strictly observant religious groups have reduced mortality and decreased rates of some diseases. Other studies have shown that prayer has beneficial therapeutic effects in large numbers of patients. A high percentage of individuals questioned on the subject felt that prayer sometimes influences recovery from illnesses, even though only half of those questioned described themselves as religious.

Unfortunately, such concepts are often not communicated between physician and patient. At a relatively early point in the patient-physician relationship, patients should mention their spiritual or religious beliefs so that physicians can be prepared to help satisfy patients' spiritual needs when and if the time for such arises.

Recommendations

1. Know the medications you take and why you are taking them.
2. Ask your doctor about side effects of prescribed medications you are given.
3. Have your doctor write down instructions.
4. Keep a list of your medications and instructions with you at all times.
5. Ask your doctor about less expensive alternatives for expensive medications.
6. Inform your doctor about your suspected medication side effects.
7. Take a list of your current medications at least yearly to your doctor and do so more often if you take numerous medications.
8. Take a spouse, relative, or friend with you to your doctor when you discuss confusing or complex treatment programs.
9. If possible, choose a single pharmacy and a personal pharmacist who is interested in providing information to you as well as in filling your prescriptions.
10. A pill container divided into daily compartments holding each day's medications is helpful for some patients, particularly the elderly.

Further Reading

The Johns Hopkins *Medical Letter*, Health After 50. September, 1994.

Alternative Medicine: Alternative to What?

Our body is a machine for living. It is organized for that, it is its nature. Let life go on in it unhindered and let it defend itself, it will do more than if you paralyze it by encumbering it with remedies.

—Leo Tolstoy, *War and Peace*

Facts

1. As many as 17 percent of adults report using herbal treatments in a given year.

2. About one-third of all Americans use some form of alternative medicine.

3. Less than one-third of patients tell their doctors that they are using some form of alternative medicine.

4. Herbal remedies, often promoted as "natural", are not necessarily harmless and can be associated with severe adverse reactions.

5. Most alternative therapies have not been evaluated through rigorously conducted scientific tests of efficacy or safety and yet may be quite expensive.

Few people would wish to pass up the opportunity to live better and longer lives because of ignorance of unusual, uncommon, or unconventional practices or therapies that could prevent or correct failings of our body systems. Familiar, conventional medical practices have indeed extended and improved life by offering cures for bacterial infections, managing or controlling heart disease, extending lifespans for those suffering from viral illnesses (e.g., AIDS), and inhibiting or slowing the growth rates of cancers. The comfort we feel with traditional medical practices lies in the fact that these practices, for the most part, are scientifically proven and supported by solid data. The successes of these practices are suggested by the extended lifespans they have fostered and the declines in certain disease entities that previously altered the qualities of those lives.

However, many individuals who are not completely satisfied with traditional medical practices have sought alternative practices, some of which have been present since ancient times. A variety of practices have been termed "alternative", including such diverse practices as:

- Acupuncture
- Homeopathy
- Herbal medicine
- Magnetic therapy
- Massage therapy
- Spiritual healing

Alternative medical practices are not commonly taught in medical schools, other than to allow for recognition of their existence, provide a forum for discussion and debate about their merits, and help students recognize potential complications related to their use. The problem with most alternative therapies is that they are highly questionable practices that have not undergone rigorously conducted tests of efficacy. Instead, alternative medicine practitioners defend their therapies by relying on testimonials, theories, anecdotes, beliefs, and endorsements that are inappropriate to the subject under discussion or are published in poor quality journals that often lack critical peer review. Alternative medicine practitioners often feel that scientific scrutiny of their remedies is just not appropriate or applicable.

Such therapies are often closely associated with certain "catch words" (e.g., "natural", "holistic", "time-tested", "complementary", or "alternative") and phrases (e.g., "stimulating the body's ability to heal itself", "mind/body interaction", "mind over matter", "power of positive thinking", "attacking the cause of disease", "treating the whole patient", "safer, nontoxic alternative", and "belief in the importance of body, mind, and spirit in health"). Some alternative medicine therapists see their roles as providers of solutions for "medicine's failures" or possibly "physician failures"; in fact, some patients have turned to alternative medicine because of instances of poor "traditional" patient/doctor or patient/medical setting relationships. It is most likely, however, that those who pursue alternative medicine practices do so in order to stay well, having had this concept suggested to them by word of mouth, books or magazines, radio and television, and more recently, the Internet. The authors have often seen older individuals who are in excellent health and have led model, healthy lifestyles begin taking absolutely unnecessary supplements.

When questioned about their good health fortune, these people often credit the supplements they take for their many good years of health rather than their many years of living healthy lifestyles, hence, the dilemma.

A complicating factor in evaluating all forms of treatment, whether they be traditional scientific, alternative, folk, or faith healing methods, is the fact that any particular treatment can at any time appear to be effective, when, in reality, it is not. This is why traditional medicine demands statistically reliable evidence from well thought out, scientifically sound studies before conclusions about a treatment's value or effectiveness can be accepted. The unexpected purported benefits that result from a broad range of unscientific therapies can be due to many, and at times complex, factors; these include:

⊙ The placebo effect – Sometimes just a subject's expectations of improvement through use of a certain treatment results in actual improvement or relief of a condition.

⊙ The healer effect – Some of today's most notable alternative medicine healers are enthusiastic, forceful individuals with charismatic personalities. They are able to captivate audiences with their seemingly endless knowledge and "factual" (though often questionable or unsubstantiated) responses. These practitioners often benefit greatly from sales of certain touted products, services, courses, and literature directed at an uncritical, unaware public.

⊙ The cooperative effect - At times, unscientific, unusual, or irrational therapies are prescribed along with worthwhile treatments such as diet, exercise, stress reduction efforts, and/or psychotherapy. Benefits from the latter rather than the former therapies may actually have brought about the desired patient improvement.

- The psychological effect – This effect can assume many forms. For example, it is commonly perceived that traditional medicine rejects religion or spirituality, which is not necessarily true. Alternative medicine practitioners who emphasize religious or spirituality concepts will no doubt benefit a segment of the population.

- The pattern of disease effect – Often a disease is self-limiting and runs its natural course, or a patient's body finally gains control of the disease process. Whatever treatment is in place at the time the disease has completed its natural course may be construed to have been the most beneficial and effective treatment method.

- The misdiagnosis effect – The original diagnosis, which may have had lethal implications and for which no known effective scientific treatment methods were available, could have been incorrect. The patient, thus, improves through use of whatever therapy was in place.

Alternative Medicine Therapies

HOMEOPATHY

Homeopathy is a practice that incorporates the concept that disease symptoms can be cured by use extremely small amounts of substances that produce similar symptoms in healthy people when taken in large amounts. Homeopathic products are so diluted that they are unlikely to have any measurable effect. They have not proven to be effective for any clinical condition and should not be used.

ACUPUNCTURE

Acupuncture therapy is based on the claim that the body's vital energy flows through channels connected to body organs and functions. Disease, it is claimed, is due to an imbalance in or interruption of flow of energy through the channels. Twirling needles in the skin at certain specific sites is supposed to reverse the imbalance or interruption.

Many theories have been suggested as to why acupuncture appears to work in some cases; endorphin production and placebo effect are commonly mentioned. Studies of this practice have been difficult to perform and are not without complications. Until more convincing studies are performed, acupuncture remains an unproven modality of treatment.

CHELATION THERAPY

A synthetic amino acid, EDTA, and other substances given intravenously to patients who seek relief from coronary artery disease, atherosclerosis, peripheral vascular disease, and a host of other major and minor illnesses.

Chelation therapy proposes to reverse the arteriosclerotic changes in coronary and extremity arteries of the body. It does not, however, appear to have any value for the suggested problem and could have potentially serious side effects.

THERAPEUTIC TOUCH

Proponents of therapeutic touch claim that a therapist can manipulate a patient's "energy field" and, thus, allow healing to occur. Energy fields, however, have never been documented, and recent studies suggest that this therapy has no value.

AYURVEDIC MEDICINE

Ayurvedic medicine is closely associated with Deepak Chopra, who may be recognized as the author of several interesting quotes, such as:

"When your actions are motivated by love, . . . the surplus energy you gather and enjoy can be channeled to create anything that you want, including limited wealth."

"They say you have to give up everything to be spiritual, get away from the world, all that junk. I satisfy a spiritual yearning without making (people) think they have to worry about God and punishment."

". . . by consciously using our awareness, we can influence the way we age biologically. . . . You can tell your body not to age."

Chopra promises "perfect health" to those who, through Ayurvedic methods, can harness consciousness as a healing force.

Chopra does quite well financially from the products he offers, including books, tapes, herbs, and aromatic oils. Critics have accused him of substituting superstition for medicine and suggest that he is delusional. The authors do not recommend Ayurvedic methods or treatments.

HERBAL MEDICINES

Herbal medicine is the most common form of alternative treatment in use. Problems have begun to arise because of herbal medicine's increasing acceptance by the public, the increased variety of products available, and the increasing number of alternative medicine practitioners prescribing them.

Herbs are processed or unprocessed plant parts, extracts, or essential oils that reach the public in a variety of forms, including tablets, capsules, teas, elixirs, and powders, and are either in pure form or are mixed with various other, often undesignated, substances. Therefore, herbs contain tremendous varieties of active chemicals whose contents and amounts can vary significantly from batch to batch. They can possess toxic as well as beneficial materials (at times, both) and have been known to contain recognized prescription compounds.

For many herbs, information related to product contents, purity, toxicity, safety, shelf-life, quality control, and interactions with other herbs, prescription medicines, and foods are unknown, incomplete, or nonexistent. Available information about herbs is often promotional and slanted, evasive in its claims, and not based on sound scientific evidence.

In the U.S., most herbal products are regulated as unpatented dietary supplements, a result of a massive lobbying effort by the health food industry that led Congress to pass the Dietary Supplement Health and Education Act (DSHEA), which classifies herbs as dietary supplements. This classification allows manufacturers of herbal products to side-step FDA rules that mandate that products claiming prevention, treatment, mitigation, or cure of disease must be treated as drugs and regulated as such; it also prevents the FDA from removing worthless ingredients from the marketplace.

If herbs were viewed as drugs, as they often, in fact, are, the FDA would oversee their manufacture to ensure safety and effectiveness, to note their possible interactions with other substances, and to designate their appropriate dosages before they were made available to the public. Additionally, the FDA would monitor their safety and effectiveness after their incorporation into medical practices.

The DSHEA also weakens the FDA's ability to protect consumers against unsubstantiated claims, allowing the herbal industry to manipulate wording so that only insinuating medical uses of a product are stated rather than actual claims of medicinal uses. This rhetoric, of course, is usually embedded in the text so that consumers will consider package labels or inserts to be as valid as those on FDA-approved product labels. In summary, the DSHEA requires no proof of efficacy or safety and sets no standards for quality control for products labeled as supplements.

The international scope of herbal product use presents still other problems. It is well recognized that herbal preparations vary considerably from country to country, and this situation further complicates evaluations of studies of herbs from different geographical locations. The effects of herbs on the body can vary tremendously, depending on the soil or climatic conditions of the areas in which they are cultivated, the methods of their storage, and the materials with which they are mixed. Chinese herbal preparations have been known to contain toxic heavy metals and, at times, other dangerous compounds and pesticides.

The approach to government oversight of product safety and quality control also varies among different countries. In Germany, for example, where herbal remedies appear to be quite popular, it has been reported that the government deliberately sets lower standards for herbal remedies than for conventional drug preparations.

Still other factors pertaining to herbal preparations are of concern. Studies have shown that herbal preparations do not always contain the ingredients indicated on their labels or that they do not contain enough of the desired herb to be effective. This makes studies of herbal products especially difficult. Some herbal preparations are so constituted that the desired active ingredient is broken down by the body's digestive system and the desired ingredient never reaches the bloodstream. Some apparently innocuous preparations, such as green tea, which has a high concentration of vitamin K, can present real problems for patients taking the blood thinner warfarin (Coumadin®). Recently, anesthesiologists have voiced concerns about patients using herbal products prior to surgery and have noted substantial changes in heart rates and blood pressures in some patients taking St. John's wort, ginko biloba, and ginseng. Anesthesiologists recommend that patients discontinue taking herbal preparations at least two to three weeks before scheduled surgeries.

Most such problems and concerns are of a type that, in the case of conventional drug manufacturing processes, would have been discovered and evaluated by the FDA, which would force manufacturers to comply with the generally accepted standards of effectiveness and safety for that preparation. Because herbal products are often real drug preparations, they should be treated as such and should undergo the same FDA scrutiny.

Recent *Associated Press* headlines herald a near fatal episode suffered by a well-known basketball star. The player suffered seizures and breathing failure after using the O-T-C herbal supplement gamma butyrolactone (GBL). According to the FDA, the product is touted for use as a sleep aid after strenuous physical activity and as a muscle recovery enhancement.

In an effort to make sense out of the voluminous, but often inadequate and usually unsubstantiated, literature about herbal preparations, the authors have summarized the best available data on several commonly used herbs (see Table 26.1). The summary notes some of the claims made for preparations as well as uses that have been suggested for them and includes their effectiveness characteristics, if these have been determined by high quality, scientific, U.S. studies performed on human subjects in appropriate numbers to make their conclusions valid. (Such studies should have taken place over adequate periods of time so as not to distort outcomes by presenting only short-term data. Appropriate studies should also have been subjected to high quality critical reviews or presented in publications that incorporate such review processes.) Considered also are quality studies of both positive and negative findings of herbal preparations in an attempt to find a consensus opinion regarding proven effectiveness characteristics.

Also considered are the presence and degree of toxic substances, if these are known, though it is impossible to consider all potential complications related to reactions with other medicines or unrecognized compounds mixed with herbal preparations. Some preparations can interfere with the effectiveness of other important prescription medications or can potentiate the actions of another drug or its toxicity.

Of concern always with use of herbal preparations is the fact that the appropriate treatment for unsuspected cancer, infection, or deficiency might be critically delayed. There is no substitute for patients communicating with personal physicians regarding any medical problems and the specific methods personally selected to manage them.

Finally, the authors provide their best recommendation regarding whether specific herbs should be incorporated into a health maintenance or life-sustaining or advancing program.

Some may argue that the authors have erected excessive barriers to the acceptance of individual herbal products. In the past, in fact, similar barriers might have prevented certain presently available drugs from being approved for public use. The authors hope, however, that the public, which is capable of learning from the past, would expect and even demand a rigid overview of products (especially those claiming or alluding to health benefits) that might find their way into our, at times, defenseless body systems.

Table 26.1 – Herbal Medicines

Medicinal Herbs	Use/Claims	Effective	Toxicity Mild	Toxicity Serious	Recommendation
Androstenedione	Boosts athletic performance	No	Yes	Yes	Avoid
Chamomile	Sedative; anti-inflammatory; wound healing	No	Yes	Yes	Avoid
Chaparral	Blood purifier; cancer cure	No	Yes	Yes	Avoid
Chondroitin, Glucosamine sulfate	Arthritis relief	Questionable	Yes	Potential	Possibly some value; better treatments available; studies in progress
Chromium picolinate	Fat burner; muscle builder	No	Yes	Yes	Avoid
Cholestin	Treats high cholesterol	Yes, as statin	Yes	Yes	Best to take quality controlled FDA-approved statin
Co-Q_{10}	Enhances energy levels cardiac support; prevents aging	No	Yes	Yes	Avoid
Creatine	Enhances performance	No	Yes	Yes	Further studies needed; will not benefit most potential users
Dong quai	Regulates menses; eases cramps	No	Yes	Yes	Avoid
DHEA	Anti-aging remedy; energy booster; retards memory loss	No	Yes	Yes	Avoid
Echinacea	Would healing; fights infections and colds	No	Yes	Yes	Avoid
Ephedra	Weight control; energy booster; asthma treatment	No	Yes	Yes	Avoid
Feverfew	Migraine prophylaxis	Yes	Yes	Yes	More studies needed

	Uses				Comments
Garlic	Prevents heart disease; lowers serum lipids; fights infection	No	Yes	Yes	Good with food preparations
Ginger	Relieves nausea and motion sickness	Yes	Yes	Unknown	Possibly useful; more studies needed
Ginko biloba	Improves mental function; slows aging; aids vascular health	No	Yes	Yes	
Ginseng	Treatment of atherosclerosis; relieves symptoms of aging; senility and cancers; aphrodisiac	No	Yes	Yes	Avoid
Goldenseal	Antidiarrheal; antiseptic	Unknown	Yes	Yes	Avoid
Green tea	Cancer prevention	Yes	Unknown	Yes	More studies needed
Kava kava	Relieves anxiety; sedative	Yes	Yes	Potential	Better studied drugs available
Melatonin	Helps with sleep and jet lag; anti-aging	Yes (sleep)	Yes	Yes	More research needed
Saw palmetto	For symptoms due to prostate enlargement	Yes	Yes	Potential	Some value shown; studies in progress
Shark cartilage	Cancer treatment; maintains healthy joints	No	Yes	Unknown	Avoid
St. John's wort	Natural antidepressant	Yes	Yes	Yes	More long-term and better studies needed; better drugs available for significant depression
Valerian	Sleep aid	Yes	Yes	Yes	Better agents available
Yohimbe	Treatment of male erectile dysfunction	Inconclusive; questionable	Yes	Yes	Take only with physician supervision

In spite of the many promises of life-enhancing and age-retarding benefits of herbal medicines or any other alternative therapies, it should become apparent that alternative medicine practices are not short-cuts to living longer and healthier lives.

Recommendations

1. If you are using herbal remedies, tell your physician about what they are.
2. Look for sound scientific data that support the value of the alternative medicine practices you are considering.
3. Research any herbal preparation you might take for toxic side effects and complications when used in combination with blood thinners.
4. Before using alternative remedies for any problem, have your personal physician determine if the problem requires medical attention.
5. Recognize that any herbal preparation might react negatively with another medication you are already taking.
6. In their book, *The Vitamin Pushers*, Barrett and Herbert (see below) strongly suggest that "the most prudent course of action is to forget about using herbs for medicinal purposes."

Further Reading

Consumer Reports, Volume 64, No. 3, March 1999.

Jaroff, Leon, What will happen to Alternative Medicine? TIME Magazine, page 77, November 8, 1999.

Newsweek, October 20, 1997.

Relman, Arnold, A Trip to Stonesville. The New Republic, December 14, 1998.

http://www.quackwatch.com

Esquire Magazine, pages 133-136, May 1999.

Barrett S., Herbert V.: *The Vitamin Pushers.* Prometheus Books, 1994.

Where the Mind Leads, the Body Will Follow

I could not at any age be content to take my place in a corner by the fireside and simply look on. Life was meant to be lived. Curiosity must be kept alive. The fatal thing is rejection. One must never, for whatever reason, turn his back on life.

-Eleanor Roosevelt

Current scientific data provide a great deal of information on extending length and quality of life. Better yet, the things we must do to achieve added years are not so difficult or unpleasant that we would need to wonder if they are worth the effort. In fact, many life extension principles were taught to us by our mothers, who admonished:

- Don't smoke.
- Eat your fruits and vegetables.
- All that greasy food isn't good for you.
- Don't sit around. Go out and play!
- Let's do some work around here.
- You're getting fat. Don't eat so much junk.
- Why do you have to drink (alcohol)?
- Drink your milk.
- Don't ever let me hear that you are using drugs.
- Get your sleep. Don't stay up all night.
- What did the doctor tell you to do?
- Why don't you find yourself some nice friends?
- Buckle-up.
- Leave the magnets on the refrigerator where they belong.

In this era of great medical advancements, physicians feel compelled to modify somewhat the wonderful words of wisdom passed on to us by our mothers. They might rephrase the messages to say:

- Don't smoke.
- Eat at least five servings of fruits and vegetables each day.
- Eat a diet low in fat, especially saturated fat and cholesterol.
- Know your blood pressure and be sure that it is normal.
- Exercise. Walk (or do some other aerobic activity) at least one-half hour each day.
- Keep your weight as close as possible to ideal for your height and build.
- Work closely with your physician on cancer screening, blood pressure control, immunizations, and vitamin, mineral, and estrogen supplements.
- Avoid more than one or two alcoholic drinks daily.
- Stay away from all illicit drugs.
- Maintain a supportive social network.
- Demand more proof of efficacy before using alternative medicine therapies.

If you follow this advice, either your mother's or your physician's, and you don't lengthen your life, notify the authors of this book and they will cheerfully refund your money.

Further Reading/References

Several outstanding sources of information on topics related to life extension are available for those interested in reading further on the subject.

BOOKS
Guide to Clinical Preventive Services, Report of the U.S. Preventive Services Task Force, 2nd ed. Williams & Wilkins 1996.

Healthy People 2000, Midcourse Review and 1995 Revisions. U.S. Department of Health and Human Services, Public Health Service.

Living Well, Staying Well: Big Health Rewards from Small Lifestyle Changes. American Heart Association and American Cancer Society, Times Books 1996.

Barrett S, Herbert V: *The Vitamin Pushers.* Prometheus Books, Amherst, N.Y. 1994.

Dietary Guidelines for Americans, 4th ed. U.S. Department of Agriculture and the U.S. Department of Health and Human Services 1994.

OTHER
Authoritative, ongoing information on subjects related to life extension can be found in the following sources:

Harvard Health Letter, 164 Longwood Ave., Boston, MA 02115.

Harvard Heart Letter, 164 Longwood Ave., Boston, MA 02115.

The Johns Hopkins *Medical Letter*: Health after 50. 550 North Broadway, Suite 1100, Johns Hopkins, Baltimore, MD 21205-2011.

Mayo Clinic *Health Letter*. 200 First Street SW, Rochester, MN 55905.

Tufts University Health & Nutrition Letter. 53 Park Place, New York, NY 10007.